Gender, Sexuality and Subjectivity

Offering a concise yet comprehensive introduction to gender theory, this thought-provoking new book aims to make an intervention into the contemporary American paradigm of thinking gender and sexuality and offers a powerful challenge to the paradigm of social constructionism.

Within each gender paradigm there are unacknowledged truths. The controversial claim of this book is that queer theory and intersectionality – and, more broadly, the social constructionist paradigm – have reached a limit. Indeed, it is possible that they are becoming regressive political gestures. However, there are possibilities of moving forward in this new area of transformation and Rousselle claims that a new logic of gender invention is opening up a new paradigm of thought.

Part of the popular Routledge Focus on Mental Health series, this book will be of immense value to students and teachers who aim to understand in a basic way some of the various main paradigms, theories, and concepts within gender and sexuality studies. It will also be an important attempt to think beyond those paradigms and theories.

Duane Rousselle, PhD, is a clinical psychoanalyst of the Lacanian orientation and Associate Professor of Sociology and Social Theory. He has published numerous books including *Jacques Lacan & American Sociology: Be Wary of the Image* (Palgrave, 2019), *Lacanian Realism: Political and Clinical Psychoanalysis* (Bloomsbury, 2018), and *Post-Anarchism: A Reader* (Pluto Press, 2012).

Routledge Focus on Mental Health

Routledge Focus on Mental Health presents short books on current topics, linking in with cutting-edge research and practice.

Titles in the series

Working with Interpreters in Psychological Therapy
The Right to be Understood
Jude Boyles and Nathalie Talbot

Rational Emotive Behaviour Therapy
A Newcomer's Guide
Walter J. Matweychuk and Windy Dryden

The Feldenkrais Method for Executive Coaches, Managers, and Business Leaders
Moving in All Directions
Paul Ogden and Garet Newell

An Evidence-based Approach to Authentic Leadership Development
Tony Fusco

Gender, Sexuality and Subjectivity
A Lacanian Perspective on Identity, Language and Queer Theory
Duane Rousselle

For a full list of titles in this series, please visit www.routledge.com/Routledge-Focus-on-Mental-Health/book-series/RFMH

Gender, Sexuality and Subjectivity

A Lacanian Perspective on Identity, Language and Queer Theory

Duane Rousselle

Routledge
Taylor & Francis Group
LONDON AND NEW YORK

First published 2020
by Routledge
2 Park Square, Milton Park, Abingdon, Oxon OX14 4RN

and by Routledge
52 Vanderbilt Avenue, New York, NY 10017

Routledge is an imprint of the Taylor & Francis Group, an informa business

British Library Cataloguing-in-Publication Data
A catalogue record for this book is available from the British Library

Library of Congress Cataloging-in-Publication Data
A catalog record for this book has been requested

ISBN: 978-0-367-44329-0 (hbk)
ISBN: 978-1-003-04481-9 (ebk)

Typeset in Times New Roman
by Apex CoVantage, LLC

Contents

Figures

Tables

1 Gender meta-theory

An in(ter)vention

The field known as 'meta-ethics' is not without its short-comings. However, its general project has been to force the discovery of truths implicit within established normative discourses. This is the profound invention of meta-ethics and the key for understanding its significance as a paradigm of thought. It is probably for this reason that meta-ethicists have proclaimed for themselves a "second-order" designation, while retroactively establishing normative ethics as restrictive and merely of the "first order" (see Mackie, 1977). Within the field of ethical philosophy, this also implies that meta-ethicists have unearthed a domain of inquiry that counts. Indeed, it is by counting to the second-order, or, in other words, by counting to 'two,' that one moves also toward the revelation of truths dormant but nonetheless determinative within normative declarations.

It is not therefore that meta-ethicists are situated somehow beyond normative ethics, and it is not as if they have surpassed the hegemonic discourse that determines them. Rather it is that meta-ethical discourses are located at the disjuncture of ethical normativity itself, by thereby revealing underlying taken-for-granted paradigmatic assumptions. Normative statements concerning the 'good' and/or 'evil' does not at all concern us because we as meta-ethicists aim to operate within the broader domain that interrogates these presuppositions by posing the following question: "whence arrive the epistemological and ontological justifications for statements concerning the 'good' and 'evil'" (see Rousselle, 2012)? It is only by asking this question that we step into the field of meta-ethics and it is only in this sense that we can claim that it involves an operation that opens up a novel discourse of the 'two.' Yes, meta-ethics is an operation that counts to 'two.' But it does not count any further.

The successful implementation of an operation that counts to 'three' requires a fundamentally different sort of invention. To count to three does not mean that one counts using the sort of logic of the "count-as-one" described by Alain Badiou ([1988] 2013), or the logic of "succession" outlined by Gottlob Frege (1960). Rather, to count to three requires the invention of another dimension of thinking, and moreover, it implies the invention of a dimension of thinking already presupposed within the restrictive conditions established by preceding truths. For this reason, I cannot claim, as I did in the past, that this is a book of meta-ethics (see Rousselle, 2012). Or, to be more precise, I cannot claim that this book is *exclusively* meta-ethical. The problem is that few of the American gender theorists – the canon of which has largely been constituted from outside sources – have learned to count beyond two, to three and/or four; and those who have are not at all aware of the profound truths that they have unearthed (much less are they aware of the various subject formations that arise as a consequence of those truth procedures).

It is through reflexive gestures (through already established paradigmatic assumptions) that serious interventions might be mapped – specifically by mapping the various truth productions and inventions. This is how we can make gender theory count again. Such an approach necessitates topological considerations that help us to orient ourselves in the labyrinth of gender theory today – or, to be more precise, since we are working now within topology: it is non-orientable, and this makes it beyond identity, language, and even beyond the queer. While working through the material that served as the support for this book, it became obvious to me that my approach – charting the dominant paradigms, theories, and concepts of gender studies – was too flat. At this point I was faced with a decision: to incorporate more material in order to satisfy the university discourse (which forever insists upon adding more and more excluded elements into a consistent and comprehensive narrative) or else to cut through university discourse, refusing its demands, by making a real intervention. Consequently, the approach of the scholar no longer cut it for me.

Inevitably, the following problem surfaced: *progressive* gender theories sometimes appeared to me to be *regressive*, and vice versa. The only way forward was to consider the ostensibly absurd possibility that my chart should be understood as a surface akin to a sheet of paper. This surface might be vectorized and the short edge twisted one hundred and eighty degrees and reattached to the other short edge. A continuous non-orientable surface was invented, which accounted for the possible movement from progressive to regressive or reactionary gender politics. I aimed to be cautious and wary of the temptation to repeat past paradigmatic comforts without also moving hastily into the new hysterical comforts of politically correct identity politics and moral posturing, which today produces a vacuum within leftist circles. Therefore, I propose to adapt Karl Marx's popular statement from his "The Eighteenth Brumaire of Louis Napoleon," which originally read "Hegel remarks somewhere that all great world-historic facts and personages appear, so to speak, twice: he forgot to add: the first time as tragedy, the second time as farce" (Marx, 1852): in the field of gender studies, victory occurs first as progress and then as regress and reaction.

It is within the context of this discovery that invention becomes exposed as a fundamental category of truth. Indeed, this book was an invention. What began as an experiment in American pedagogy (for courses in the sociology of gender and sexuality at Grand Valley State University in Grand Rapids, Michigan) resulted in the invention of a new teaching strategy. Scribbles upon a few sheets of paper – various formulae, charts, diagrams, and so on – were placed upon the podium in front of me. American students are a product of the discourse that compels them, and that discourse is none other than the 'capitalist discourse,' the new, fifth, master discourse discovered by Jacques Lacan (see Rousselle, 2019). It is a discourse that demands modules, slides, pre-established chunks of knowledge designed only for the purposes of plugging up the anxiety of thinking. It is a demand that is instigated by an environment which exemplifies pragmatist ideology, and which mutates the traditional discourse of the university (ibid.). I invented a new teaching method – oriented by scribbles – as an attempt to frustrate these demands.

It was this frustration of demand that moved me toward an obscure interrogation of gender studies, toward an examination of the broad tendency of theory itself. It is at this level that I entered what the American sociologist George Ritzer has named "meta-theory" (Ritzer, 2007). It is the word 'paradigm,' by which I mean to describe the zone in which unconscious presuppositions develop into theoretical orientations, that nonetheless introduces further confusion: what is a meta-theory and how is it different from a paradigm? Any discussion of meta-theory must be connected to a discussion of its paradigmatic assumptions, and this is missing (and yet most encouraged) in most meta-theoretical analyses. There I stood in front of American students, with the demands of capitalist discourse – with its incredible sense of urgency and its movement from one 'chunk' of knowledge to another so as to reduce theory only to its "cash-value" (Rousselle, 2019) – and I offered an obstacle or a barrier: an obscure silence laced with topological significance.

The anxiety of thinking produced in me stuttering and stammering, and there, within the classroom, I often fell silent. But this is precisely the antidote to the chaos of capitalist discourse. It was my aim to demonstrate to these students the profound anxiety of thinking, the likes of which were once described by Søren Kierkegaard, who wrote that "learning to be anxious so as not to be ruined either by never having been in anxiety or by sinking into it, . . . whoever has learned to be anxious in the right way has learned the ultimate" (Kierkegaard, 2015). This saving virtue one learns courageously, as an appropriate subject formation vis-à-vis truth. Capitalist university discourse does not entirely destroy the possibility of adopting this courageous subject formation, although that is what it certainly intends to do.

I wish therefore to thank those students who refused to flee from the anxiety of thinking, and who received, whether they were aware of it or not, the reward of invention. Together we crossed the Rubicon that separates the real and the body of knowledge that intends to govern it, and if only for the moment, we demonstrated that within the urgency of the capitalist university, it is indeed possible to burst the bubble that separates the classroom from the rest of the world.

References

Badiou, Alain. [1988] (2013) *Being & Event* (Oliver Feltham, Trans.). London: Bloomsbury Books.

Frege, Gottleb. (1960) *The Foundations of Arithmetic: A Logico-Mathematical Enquiry into the Concept of Number* (J. L. Austin, Trans.). New York: Harper & Brothers.

Kierkegaard, Søren. (2015) "Anxiety as Saving through Faith," in *The Concept of Anxiety: A Simple Psychologically Oriented Deliberation in View of the Dogmatic Problem of Hereditary Sin*. New York, NY: Liveright.

Mackie, John L. (1977) *Ethics: Inventing Right and Wrong*. New York: Penguin Books.

Marx, Karl. (1852) "The Eighteenth Brumaire of Louis Bonaparte," As Retrieved on May 29th, 2019 from <www.marxists.org/archive/marx/works/1852/18th-brumaire/>

Ritzer, George. (2007) "Metatheory," in *The Blackwell Encyclopedia of Sociology*. Wiley Online Library.

Rousselle, Duane. (2012) *After Post-Anarchism*. San Francisco, CA: Repartee Books.

Rousselle, Duane. (2019) *Jacques Lacan and American Sociology: Be Wary of the Image*. London, England: Palgrave Books.

2 Theory as an antidote to chaos

Theory orients us within the labyrinth of the social world by situating our naïve taken-for-granted assumptions within an appropriate symbolic apparatus. A distinction, then: theory must be distinguished to some extent from its underlying paradigmatic framework. Whereas paradigms consist of raw unconscious presuppositions, theory merely attempts to navigate and map the terrain of those same presuppositions. This is why we might relate this definition of a paradigm to that of the 'symbolic unconscious' described at length by members of the World Association of Psychoanalysis. At the center of the Freudian discovery, as its fundamental truth production, there was for a long time an exploration of the symbolic unconscious: the unconscious must be interpreted, deciphered, or translated into a meaningful system of signifiers, a coherent and consistent body of knowledge or a narrative concerning the social environment.

The work of theory is often to reveal latent signifiers which, when taken together, constitute our apparently spontaneous opinions or clusters of knowledge. These opinions or knowledges in turn move us and orient us in our social environments. From this perspective, then, a body (*any* body whatsoever) is formed as a meaningful body, a textured body, as a body inscribed by signifiers. The body is a zone of signification. Thus, the body, when viewed from within the social constructionist paradigm, is always one that is constructed from the raw materials of language, and this is what constitutes the cornerstone of the social constructionist paradigm within sociology. Yet this approach avoids another altogether more provocative possibility: the 'real unconscious,' which confronts us as a body of confusions, ambiguities, obscurities, rather than the fleeting comforts of meaningful explanations.

A paradigm is related to the symbolic unconscious such that if one thinks that something is true, that it is beyond debate, or if one holds an unshakable conviction, then one is all the more operating within the set of those unacknowledged paradigmatic assumptions. The more obvious an explanation given by an individual seems to be to us, the more anchored it is to an underlying paradigmatic presupposition. For example, there is the often repeated 'go-to' answer held by people that gender is simply equivalent to sex and that it has everything to do with our innate biological constitution. This is one of the key paradigmatic assumptions: gender is sex is biology. This position has the virtue of making matters simple so that we do not have to engage with the confusions or inconveniences of real sexuality or gender. If we affirm this position, we also have the advantage of simply moving on with our lives, of moving forward in our everyday discussions without having to be bogged down by the anxieties of careful reflection.

Within contemporary American society, there is the following paradigmatic assumption: the world is out there, external to the individual, and it is an intelligible or meaningful world. Thus, that world can be understood empirically, objectively. The role of the sociologist or 'social scientist' is to somehow see the world for what it really is, without any ideological distortions or bias. We often expect from the sociologist the same attitude that we expect from the American news network Fox News: a 'no spin' zone, a world free of bias, a world of cold facts. And yet, precisely when one presents oneself as being situated within the no spin zone, one becomes all the more susceptible to accusations of bias. Why? On the one hand, we are supposed to remove our biases, step outside of our ideologies, detach ourselves from our prejudices, and just be attentive to the world as it is; yet on the other hand, whenever we do this we end up having to entertain the possibility proposed by Kellyanne Conway during her *Meet the Press* interview in early 2017: there are "alternative facts," a world where "facts are not facts."

It is as if we are trying to remove the various distortions that stand in between us and our ascertaining of the social world, between us and reality, between the 'fake news' and the truth. In other words, even the political left today – the harbingers of the 'social constructionist' paradigm within popular culture – seem to want a no spin version of the social world. We imagine that ideology consists of something like a pair of sunglasses that distorts one's vision of the social world, and yet as Slavoj Zizek correctly claimed many years ago, ideology exists precisely when we take off the sunglasses (Zizek, 2013). We therefore have to reverse our way of thinking: it is only when we put on the sunglasses of theory – the supposedly distorting lenses of theory – that we can see a paradigm for what it is: these distortions are already present in the fabric of reality itself.

In other words, we should begin with the assumption that a paradigm is always present and that we cannot so easily step outside of our paradigmatic assumptions. Theory functions to introduce a lens, to mediate us from the outside world, so that we can selectively form some impression about that world. Our job is therefore to put on theory sunglasses. When I was young there existed a suitable version of this: red sheets of paper with nonsensical scribbles upon them, accompanied by red 'decoder glasses.' When you wear the red decoder glasses you are suddenly able to discern shapes, figures, and text within the chaotic scribbles etched upon the paper. This is the role of theory: we require the correct theories to make sense of the scribbles that pervade and permeate the social world and indeed, our situated and gendered bodies. Good theory can help us decide the hidden, unconscious, or latent presuppositions that govern our understandings of the social world. It is only in this way that ideology liberates rather than imprisons us.

When we begin with the assumption that gender is biological – that gender *is* sex – it is clear that we lack the proper decoder glasses to understand the meaning that structures our assumption. It is by attacking this naïve position that proclaims that gender is simply biological, that sociology and gender studies today plots a course. Indeed, we see that it is the premise of the popular textbook *Gender Reckonings: New Social Theory and Research* edited by Raewyn Connell (2018). This textbook shall be used, among other resources, in my own study you have before you. My conviction is that theory itself needs to be updated. The problem is that old theories are no longer orienting us in the new world; we have reached an impasse and the criticality of gender studies has been blunted: "[w]e think the time has arrived for a fresh look at these questions, and a critical rethinking of current theory" (ibid., 2018: 1). On this point, I am in agreement: today more than ever we require a return to theory. We need to sharpen our edges and fold them back in upon one another.

At the minimum, a good theory requires concepts. But as the editor of the aforementioned book, *Gender Reckonings*, explains, "a lot of what passes for social analysis of gender is conceptually weak. Hasty gestures toward 'gender norms,' 'social constructionism,' or 'stereotypes' do not explain much" (ibid., 2018: 1). I take here the etymological connection in the word 'theory,' which carries a sense of 'viewing' or 'seeing' as if from a distance. It is the distance of theory, the distance which theory affords, that permits the sociologist or gender scholar a reflexive thinking about gender paradigms, without which there is only the taken-for-granted ideological position that *gender is sex is biology is unchanging is a fact*. Indeed, the problem with those who do not position themselves within theory is that they begin with the assumption of there being a factual knowledge, against which there are only the accounts of those who promulgate 'fake news.' They believe themselves outside of the apparatus of ideology.

However, there is also the alternative fact that theory itself permits one to become stupid in the face of one's already established paradigmatic assumptions. Take, for example, the narrative offered to us by Charles Baudelaire, as a toddler who with careful artistry witnessed his father dressing: the boy "looked at the arm muscle, the colour tones of the skin tinged with rose and yellow, and the bluish network of veins, . . . need I say that, today, the child is a famous painter" (Baudelaire, 1964: 8). In other words, the child was stupid (whereby stupid implies that one is once again 'stunned' or 'amazed' by the world). Or, put another way, to be like a child is to no longer allow oneself to take for granted pre-established bodies of meaning. It is to no longer take the body for granted. During this period, the child looks at the world with fresh eyes and complete ignorance before he grows up to know quite a bit (perhaps too much).

The task we have before us is therefore to be stupid again, to make new choices about what is true and what is false, to unearth the presuppositions that have structured our engagement with the social world and with gender and sexuality, and to consider the alternatives. I refer to one such set of presuppositions as the 'essentialist paradigm.' For now, we may simplify our definition of the essentialist paradigm to the following: for those who adhere to these taken-for-granted truths, there is the belief that gender is tied to a set of characteristics that are unchanging. Gender is essentially tied to certain attributes, qualities, properties, which assist us in forming a conviction concerning gender assignment. The best example that we have of this paradigm is that of 'biological essentialism,' championed by medicine, science, and many religious schools of thought. The core assertion is that the body is from birth identified by certain biological markers (e.g., penis, vagina, breasts, testosterone, and so on) that not only indicates but also preserves the meaning of the gendered body throughout time.

I shall provide a provisional definition for the second paradigm, the one that still remains dominant in American universities, namely 'social constructionism.' For now, I claim only that the social constructionist paradigm begins with the presupposition that gender is a system of meanings transmitted from the social environment into each individual who inhabits that environment, such that these individuals endlessly confirm and negotiate the meanings or scripts throughout their everyday lives. This paradigm is a broad one and it includes theories that we shall consider in later chapters, including 'intersectionality,' 'Marxist feminisms,' 'queer theories,' 'post-structuralism,' and so on. My claim is that the social constructionist paradigm – with all of its politically correct language and progressive political overtones – has today reached an impasse in America. We have, therefore, what is outlined in Table 2.1.

Table 2.1 Major paradigms and theories in gender theory

Paradigm	*Theory*
Essentialist	Biological/Trumpian
Social constructionist	Intersectionality theories Marxist feminisms Queer theories Post-structuralism

That there are impasses to social constructionism does not imply that we should immediately abandon it. It implies rather that we dig deep also into its presuppositions so as to reveal its various truth productions and inventions. Today in America, social constructionism is being challenged from within and from without: gender and women's studies departments are gradually being defunded, popular culture has attacked what they perceive as its 'social justice warrior' tendency and its obsession with political correctness, and the president of the United States, Donald Trump, seems to have taken a reactionary position by proclaiming once again that gender is defined by biological markers. These are dark times. We no longer know how to move forward, so we cling to and dramatize the only paradigm that we know. Imagine yourself as a sailor on a ship floating in the dark sea. We see ahead of us, thankfully, a small light, a beacon. We cannot move in a straight line toward it, and yet we try. This is the beacon that I am looking at: it is an opportunity to reorient ourselves in the darkness. We cannot move straight toward our goal because the waves come crashing at us. But nonetheless, we try. As we approach the beacon, we realize that it is another ship that is about to crash into us.

This is what the future shows to us, much like the infamous painting of *Angelus Novus* by Paul Klee, as described so eloquently by Walter Benjamin in his "On the Concept of History":

> An angel is depicted there who looks as though he were about to distance himself from something which he is staring at. . . . His face is turned towards the past. . . . [H]e sees . . . unceasingly piles [of] rubble on top of rubble and hurls it before his feet. He would like to pause for a moment so fair, to awaken the dead and to piece together what has been smashed. But a storm is blowing from Paradise, it has caught itself up in his wings and is so strong that the Angel can no longer close them. The storm drives him irresistibly into the future, to which his back is turned, while the rubble-heap before him grows sky-high. That which we call progress, is *this* storm.
>
> (Benjamin, 1940)

This is how we should understand the project before us: the distance we achieve as we move from the one paradigm to the next comes also with a vantage point to see the rubble of the truth that preceded us, and yet with each truth production there is yet another push from the wind of progress and yet another crash into the seas of the paradigms that preceded us. Nonetheless, we try.

References

Baudelaire, Charles. (1964) *The Painter of Modern Life and Other Essays* (J. Mayne, Trans., Ed.). London: Phaidon Press.

Benjamin, Walter. (1940) *On the Concept of History* (Dennis Redmond, Trans.). As Retrieved on May 11th, 2019 from <www.marxists.org/reference/archive/benjamin/1940/history.htm>

Connell, Raewyn. (2018) *Gender Reckonings: New Social Theory and Research*. New York: NYU Press.

Zizek, Slavoj. (2013) *The Perverts Guide to Ideology* (Sophie Fiennes, Dir.). Zeitgeist Films.

3 Thinking gender as a Marxist

Foundational ideas

In this chapter I will provide a basic overview of the Marxist position. In Chapter 2, I made a distinction between 'paradigm' and 'theory.' This distinction does not imply an opposition because theories are always situated within or anchored to their respective overarching paradigms. In other words, theories are ways of navigating and making good use of the assumptions that compel us to think and act according to our various determinations. For this reason, it is incorrect to claim – and some theorists do – that theory gives us a special vantage point from which to step outside of our unconscious determinations. It is quite often precisely the opposite: theory permits us to step directly into them, assume them, and to take responsibility for them. Theory brings us deeper inside the paradigm from which we seek to escape, and this, paradoxically, is the only way to take ethical responsibility: paradigms can determine us from behind our back or else they can be directed to productive ends.

When we claim that a paradigm includes all of the statements and declarations that we take for granted about the social world, this also implies that it includes all of the questions that we think are the important ones to ask. Even our questions therefore lack the innocence and naivety that we often attribute to them. The questions we ask always demand a particular response from our interlocutor. Jacques Lacan went so far as to claim that questions presuppose an answer that one has already accepted. We cannot get outside of our own heads! This reminds me of the sort of statement made by Saint John of the Cross in his *Ascent of Mount Carmel:* "understanding can understand naught save that which is contained within" (Saint John of the Cross, 2006), or the lesson of Jacques-Alain Miller many decades later that "one only understands what one thinks one already knows . . . one never understands anything but a meaning whose satisfaction or comfort one has already felt" (Miller, xxvi). The final word on this must go to Jacques Lacan:

> Questions interest me very much. They interest me very much in the sense that every question is only ever formed on the basis of an answer. That's for certain. We only ask questions when we already have the answer. This seems to me to very much limit the scope of the question.
>
> (Lacan as cited by Hewitson, 2014)

What could this mean? It implies that even there, where we most believe ourselves to have stepped outside of our biases, during our eager and selfless mode of questioning, we are in fact all the more trapped by the biases we thought we escaped. The questions we ask about gender, the questions we consider to be the important ones within the field of gender theory, or within sociology, are already limited in scope; even our questions are not innocent. This is why somebody like Slavoj Zizek has claimed that the crucial task of philosophy is not to come up with answers to all of the world's problems (there are so many better situated fields) but rather to demonstrate that the questions we are asking about the world are themselves already strategies of misdirection, that they are already inhibited by the paradigmatic assumptions made upon the pervasive stage of ideology (Zizek, 2019). Theory is therefore novel only in the sense that it shows us what we have already presupposed but refused to consciously accept. It reveals to us the unpleasant truths that determine and structure our various ways of thinking, interpreting, and acting in the world. It is for this reason that I use the words paradigm and ideology as synonyms, but also because the former term is much more accepted within sociology departments in America.

I suggest three components for any definition of ideology: first, ideology is unconscious; second, ideology is always a way of constituting a body of knowledge; and third, ideology has no outside. I draw as support for this tripartite definition the theory of Louis Althusser, a French Marxist who once wrote that "ideology has little to do with consciousness – it is profoundly unconscious" (1971). However, I also insist, with Althusser, that ideology consists, for the most part, of symbolic elements that form an unconscious and therefore decipherable body (of knowledge): once again, ideology provides us with pre-fabricated answers about chaotic reality. When we discuss knowledge, we do so always with a discursive definition provided by Jacques Lacan: a body, in its imaginary dimension, is always a linkage of S1 and S2, which, in non-technical terms, are two particles of language conjoined into a chunk of knowledge. But this leaves still to be explored the third ideological characteristic, that there is no outside. I will work my way, in this chapter, toward a satisfying definition.

The problem is that Marx himself did not have a sophisticated theory of ideology. We know, for example, his famous and oft-quoted statement from *The German Ideology:* "The ideas of the ruling class are in every epoch the ruling ideas" (Marx, 2019). Ideology is always a mode of domination and may very well be the word to describe the *fact* of domination. Marx continued, "[t]he ruling ideas are nothing more than the ideal expression of the dominant material relationships, the dominant material relationships grasped as ideas; hence of the relationships which make the one class the ruling one, therefore, the ideas of its dominance" (ibid.). Marx's position was that real reality is forever eclipsed by the ideas of the dominating class, and this, as it were, is the function of ideology. Ideology presents ideas to us as if they were rendered by a *camera obscura*, that is, in inverted form. Rather than present the antagonism at the heart of the social bond, American ideology today presents a series of false equivalences.

Louis Althusser introduced some new insights and thereby extended Marx's more basic theory of ideology. Marx's more simplistic theory described the "means of production" as comprising those essential tools that are required for the extraction of surplus value by the bourgeoisie (e.g., shovels, conveyor belts, and so on) out of the proletariat. These tools were under the ownership of the dominating class, and this was their crucial advantage over the subordinate working class. However, the most important of these tools are workers themselves: workers are also a part of the "means of production" because of their labour potential and power. It is because of the prior advantage of ownership (e.g., especially of the means of production) that the bourgeoisie are able to purchase the labour power of the proletariat. The bourgeoisie are the class who are situated in such a way within the social bond that they are best able to reinvest and gain extra exponential economic surplus.

In American sociology today, we consider Marx's position to be within the scope of a 'conflict theory.' Conflict theories assert that at the heart of the social bond there is a fundamental conflict. In the case of Marxism, the conflict exists between the bourgeoisie and the proletariat (minimally), and the consequent rift situates the two differently within a general ideology or worldview. For example, there are the following two infamous Marxist formulae: $M_1 \rightarrow C \rightarrow M_2$ and $C_1 \rightarrow M \rightarrow C_2$. The first formula designates bourgeois logic, whereby money exists in "time one" as "M_1," which, in "time two," may be used to purchase commodities, "C," including, essentially, labour power, which, finally, in "time three" produces profit, "M_2." The second formula designates proletariat logic whereby one begins with one's labour power only, which is sold as a commodity, "C_1," to the bourgeoisie to generate money, "M," which in "time three" may be used to purchase commodities that would fulfil basic needs, "C_2."

The problem that inevitably arises is this: how is it that the essential tools required for production remain operative throughout time? The answer that inevitably emerges: through endless reinvestments. Shovels become blunted and will need to be replaced, trucks will require repairs, and so on. Yet people also get worn out and they, just like any other of the essentialist commodities, must be the recipients of reinvestments. One must invest in the continual improvement of the most essential commodity, the worker. It is for this reason that Louis Althusser introduced a theory of the "reproduction of the means of production." The bourgeoisie shall invest in the proletariat in numerous ways: by granting them 'sick days,' short breaks for lunch and replenishment, healthcare, bonuses, wage/salary increases, and so on. No doubt, this explains why philanthropists invest in community projects such as hospitals and schools. From the strict perspective of ideology, it is to ensure that the worker and his children continually return to the factory gate each day and therefore continue to be resigned to their fate within capitalist production. Althusser wrote that all of this "enables the wage earner to present himself again at the factory gate the next day – and every further day God grants him" (Althusser, 1971).

There is a further way that the bourgeoisie can ensure the reproduction of the 'means of reproduction': through ideology, or in other words, through culture. Ideology is merely the name we give to the political and economic project implied in a paradigm. For Althusser, there is no outside to ideology. It was a theory of ideology carefully worked in correspondence to (and in proximity to) Jacques Lacan's psychoanalytic theories. Ideology is unconscious, claimed Althusser. Yet it is also a type of knowledge. I take an example from Slavoj Zizek, who for his part, extracted it and reworked it from the former American Secretary of Defence, Donald Rumsfeld (2003). Rumsfeld was discussing the rationale for the war in Iraq and he claimed the following: there are *known knowns* (things that you consciously know), there are *known unknowns* (things that you consciously know that you do not know), and there are *unknown unknowns* (things that you do not even know that you do not know).

There are words on this page, and *I know that I know it*. These are the 'known knowns.' There are also a certain number of words in this book, and without counting them *I know that I do not know* how many words there are. This is the point, *I know that I do not know it*. These are the 'known unknowns.' Finally, there are the things that *I do not even know that I do not know*. Possibly, these are the evil things, such as weapons of mass destruction. In other words, they are the 'unknown unknowns.' Years later Rumsfeld realized that he missed one further combination: 'unknown knowns.' These are the things that *I didn't know that I (already) knew*. He said the following: "[t]here are known knowns. There are known unknowns. There are unknown unknowns. But there are also unknown knowns, that is to say the things you think you know that it turns out you did not" (Rumsfeld, 2016). What Rumsfeld did not realize was that his final definition still radically missed the proper interpretation of the 'unknown knowns,' which has no other explanation than what we have been calling until now a 'paradigm' or our 'symbolic unconscious.'

Finally, we turn to the claim that "there is no outside to ideology." Ideology is also immersive. This does not mean that there cannot be various ideologies (in the plural), each with their own distinctive content, each with their own epistemological assertions. It means rather that ideology is itself a *form* within which finite systems of knowledge – chunks of knowledge, in the contemporary American context – may be present. For example, there may be different gender ideologies that are constructed to provide answers to questions concerning the relations between the sexes, the significance and meaning of various identities, and so on. It is not that the social world is approached through various distortions of reality but rather that reality itself is a distortion that requires theoretical elaboration, and this is how we should interpret Althusser's expression that "ideology represents the imaginary relationship of individuals to their real conditions of existence" (Althusser, 1971).

Those who claim to be outside of ideology are by definition all the more inside. Althusser wrote:

> [T]hose who are in ideology believe themselves by definition outside ideology: one of the effects of ideology is the practical *denegation* of the ideological character of ideology by ideology: ideology never says, 'I am ideology.' It is necessary to be outside ideology . . . to be able to say: I am in ideology . . . I was in ideology.
>
> (Althusser, 1971)

This is why the topological structure of ideology is none other than that of a Klein bottle (which, incidentally, consists of two Mobius strips – a right-pass and a left-pass – brought together to remove all edges). The Klein bottle is such that as you pass through its canal, through its hole, you move further inward before finding your way to the true outside. Conversely, it is only by moving further outward that you can find your way inside of the Klein bottle. This is a nice corrective to the traditional narrative of Plato's cave whereby the movement is presumed to go from inside of the cave – inside of a hole – toward the outside. In naïve terms: one is supposed to move from ideology toward enlightenment, from inside to outside. This simplistic topology misses the possibility of the existence of spaces of 'ext-imacy,' and, moreover, the allegory positions the philosopher as the enlightened *one*, free from confinement, free from the prison cell. I would like to provide a counterpoint.

A similar allegory is presented to us by the Quran, Surah 18, *al-Kahf*, translated into English as "The Cave." It teaches of seven individuals who abandoned the terrifying freedoms of the pagan city (e.g., the freedom to worship any God, any idol, etc.) to pursue their more dogmatic religious convictions. They took refuge inside of a cave and brought along with them a dog to guard its entrance. This is not the philosopher's cave of eventual enlightenment; it is a paradoxical cave inside of which the sleepers were able to tranquilize the excessiveness of their freedoms. Indeed, the Quran indicates to us that the sleepers were most awake precisely when they fell asleep inside of the cave: "you would have thought them awake, while they were asleep" (Surah Al-Kahf 18:18). Does this not indicate to us that it is paradoxically by connecting to our dreams or ideologies that we become most enlightened, or that it is paradoxically by finding our cave that we can reach a purer freedom in our voluntary submission to the unconscious?

There have been many variations of the Platonic allegory. For example, McKenzie Wark once introduced the following amendment to students of cultural studies at Trent University: when the individual leaves the cave he finds himself inside of yet another cave. Although this appears to be a clever twist on the allegory, it nonetheless only returns us to the initial problem of there being "no outside to ideology." The Lacanian twist is therefore the best in that it suggests that the cave has none other than the topological structure of a Klein bottle. This, finally, is how we should read Althusser's claim that the only way outside of ideology is to burrow oneself within it. It is the darkness of the cave rather than the light of outside freedoms to which we must today turn our attention. Giorgio Agamben contends that this is what it means to be truly contemporary:

> The ones who can call themselves contemporary are only those who do not allow themselves to be blinded by the lights of the century, and so manage to get a glimpse of the shadows in those lights, of their intimate obscurity. . . . The contemporary

> is the person who perceives the darkness of his time as something that concerns him, as something that never ceases to engage him. Darkness is something that – more than any light – turns directly and singularly toward him. The contemporary is the one whose eyes are struck by the beam of darkness that comes from his own time.
>
> (Agamben, 2009: 45)

If the dream seems to most as a flight from reality, then one should return for a moment to an argument originally presented to us by Sigmund Freud: it is the liar who we can most trust with the truth. If, for example, an individual declares "I always tell the truth," we know very well that we should be even more careful and suspicious of them. We are already in the presence of a blatant liar, since to be human is to lie at some point in our lives. Yet on the other hand, if one proclaims "I am a liar!" then we can be sure that there is some degree of truth in their statement: it is within the darkness of their lie that we can be sure of there being some consistency or truth.

And it is the same today with the American obsession with 'fake news,' 'no spin zones,' and 'alternative facts.' When the president of the United States describes the fake news machines, he deliberately exempts himself (and Fox News) from that designation and thereby renews his trick. It is precisely by exposing the truth of 'fake news' that he is able to position himself as somehow outside of the effects of the fake news machines such as the *New York Times*, *Washington Post*, and so on. Yet this move is an ideological gesture par excellence! Ideology, spin, bias, etc., are not reserved for *other* people. It is the work of ideology to claim that it is only *others* who are not immune to its effects.

For a long time within classical Marxism, gender was considered to be a distraction from the class struggle. It was thought that gender was an ideological distortion of a more fundamental class antagonism. If on the one hand, one is supposed to focus on issues of 'pay equity,' 'gender discrimination' in the workplace, and so on, so that in the final instance the workplace becomes more fair but also more acceptable to the worker (and therefore more of an uncontestable site of exploitation), then on the other hand, those who refuse to consider the workplace as the fundamental site of exploitation are often viewed by classical Marxists as being among those situated outside of proletarian consciousness. They are considered ideological for this reason. It is Marxism which here reveals itself as an ideologically driven project.

Marxist feminists, such as Nancy Fraser, maintain that gender conflict is anchored to a fundamental class antagonism. For example, she stated the following:

> I think the days of putting feminism against . . . Marxism are over. . . . Some report that the problem is that Marx failed to actually think systematically about this question and to really theorize it and conceptualize it as a major dimension of capitalist society. . . . Marx would have agreed that socialism cannot simply mean socialized ownership of the means of production. It also has to mean collectivization of housework and social reproduction.
>
> (Fraser, 2018)

For Nancy Fraser and others, it is simply a question of extending the basic presuppositions of Marxist conflict theory. There is nonetheless a reticence regarding drawing out and exploring the consequences of any encounter of Marxist analyses with feminism or gender theory. There has been a refusal for many decades to position gender as its own relatively autonomous site of conflict or antagonism. But as we all know, today's Marxist gender theorists are actively seeking to articulate gender and patriarchy as relatively autonomous sites of antagonism that nonetheless intersect with and exacerbate class conflict.

References

Agamben, Giorgio. (2009) "What Is the Contemporary?," in *What Is an Apparatus? And Other Essays* (David Kishik & Stefan Pedatella, Trans.). Stanford, CA: Stanford University Press.

Althusser, Louis. (1971) "Ideology and Ideological State Apparatuses," As Retrieved on May 11th, 2019 from <www.marxists.org/reference/archive/althusser/1970/ideology.htm>

Fraser, Nancy. (2018) "Nancy Fraser: Marx and Feminism," [Video] As Retrieved on May 12th, 2019 from <www.youtube.com/watch?v=w0448ptJ4Ic>

Hewitson, Owen. (2014) "The Value of Stupid Questions," *LacanOnline*. As Retrieved on May 11th, 2019 from <www.lacanonline.com/2014/03/lessons-from-lacans-practice-everyday-psychoanalysis-from-the-classroom-to-the-boardroom-iv/>

Marx, Karl. (2019) *The German Ideology*. As Retrieved on May 11th, 2019 from <www.marxists.org/archive/marx/works/1845/german-ideology/ch01b.htm>

Miller, Jacques-Alain. (1990) "Micro-Scopia," in *Television: A Challenge to the Psychoanalytic Establishment* (Jeffrey Mehlman, Trans., Joan Copjec, Ed.). New York: W. W. Norton & Company.

Rumsfeld, Donald. (2003) "The Unknown Knowns," [Video] As Retrieved on May 11th, 2019 from <www.youtube.com/watch?v=nAnKdq5Yty8>

Saint John of the Cross. (2006) *The Ascent of Mount Carmel* (David Lewis, Trans., Benedict Zimmerman, Ed.). Whitefish, MT: Kessinger Publishing.

Zizek, Slavoj. (2019) "The Task of Philosophy Isn't to Solve Problems," [Video] As Retrieved on May 11th, 2019 from <www.youtube.com/watch?v=hJbUFxZvWWY>

4 The social construction of gender

The case of queer theory

In Chapter 3, I tried to provide a basic overview of the debate between classical Marxism and feminism. Within the classical Marxist perspective, the following possible claims seem to have been made:

1 The class struggle – the struggle between the bourgeoisie and the proletariat – is the most fundamental and therefore the only struggle of interest for our analysis because it is the battle that permits one class to continually extract surplus value and to reinvest. This was what the following formula illustrated: $M_1 \rightarrow C \rightarrow M_2$. In other words, class struggle is the central conflict around which all other struggles revolve. Other struggles are either distractions or else are reducible to the primary site of class conflict. Consequently, any sort of gender conflict will be considered an ideological distortion or distraction. For this position, discussions of gender are ideological and therefore serve the interests of ideological state apparatuses (legitimization of the inherent class conflict at the base).

A historical example will sufficiently demonstrate the strength of this discourse for those who uphold it. During the Spanish civil war, between 1936 and 1939, there were tactical alliances formed among the various radical militants. These militants were usually Marxists or anarchists in their various orientations. Of course, there was also intense infighting among these militant factions. A wonderful study conducted by Martha Ackelsberg (1991) demonstrated that there was within the anti-capitalist and anti-fascist movement the discovery of another axis of oppression: women desired to join the men to fight against capitalism and fascism, but their efforts were thwarted. Ackelsberg wrote: "In 1936, groups of women in Madrid and Carcelona founded *Mujeres Libres*, an organization dedicated to the liberation of women from their 'enslavement . . . as women and as producers'" (Ackelsberg, 1991: 21).

Put another way, the *Mujeres Libres*, or the "Free Women of Spain," were fighting a 'class war' but were also, alongside and at the same time as the class war, were involved in a gender war. The conflict therefore occurred for them in two dimensions: capitalist exploitation and fascist impositions, as well as patriarchal domestication.

2 Another related discourse claimed that women themselves were involved in the "reproduction of the 'means of production'" and were therefore ideological in character. Whereas the former position claimed that gender conflict was a distraction, this claims rather that women themselves, because of their situated identity, are by necessity ideological. This discourse might even be extended to include the more contemporary one, which claims that any discussion of 'non-traditional' gender categories are always forms of ideological distortion from the central concern of class-struggle and revolution.

In any case, the classical Marxist position has been that those who partake in unpaid or invisible labour are unable to achieve proletarian consciousness. The claim is that they cannot become aware of their exploitation and oppression because they are not directly the objects of surplus extraction for the bourgeoisie. Thus, Marx's famous description of the 'class-in-itself' and the 'class-for-itself' – whereby the goal is to move from the former to the latter, from 'ideological consciousness' to what I would name 'consciousness of ideology' – demonstrates precisely that the turn toward class-consciousness, toward being a class-for-itself, depends essentially upon membership in that class. This, nonetheless, is a topological argument concerning the location of a set of individuals within the social bond. But it is, however, a limited perspective.

3 Finally, there is a more contemporary position that fundamentally reorients the discussion. If the first position claimed that gender conflict is ideological, and the second claimed that women themselves are ideological, then, finally, there has been the redevelopment, within and alongside of classical Marxian theories, of a newer theory of gender that claims that gender is a relatively independent or to borrow a phrase from Althusser, "relatively autonomous," site of power and conflict. This perspective breaks from the two preceding ones by rejecting the possibility that (1) the study of gender conflict is an ideological distraction, and (2) women (and by implication non-traditional genders) are inherently ideological. The proposal is simply that gender conflict is just as important as class conflict and that neither shall take priority over the other.

We might formulate the classical Marxist position in the following way: *Classical Marxist Position == Class Conflict (Gender Conflict)*. This formula indicates that in the classical Marxist discourse (an older position historically, but as a discourse, it nonetheless lingers throughout the present), discussions of 'gender conflict' were subsumed within the overarching fundamental 'class conflict.' The contemporary position within Marxist thinking on gender may be illustrated in the following way: *Contemporary Conflict Theory = (Class Conflict ( ) Gender Conflict)*. Within this formula, contemporary conflict theory is defined by the study of the intersectionality (e.g., the 'logical biconditional') as well as the exclusivity (e.g., the 'exclusive or') of the two sets of theory. Put simply, one studies the intersection of the two zones of conflict while nonetheless remaining committed to independent observations.

It seems to me that it was this final, third perspective that was transformative for contemporary American sociological inquiries into gender. Suddenly, during the second-wave period of feminist movement from the 1960s until the 1990s, 'socialist feminists' and 'Marxist feminists' stopped presuming that one conflict was the most important or fundamental. This paradigmatic assumption of the importance of studying the intersection as well as the independence of the two conflicts continued to increase in influence. However, to be very clear, this was not the position demonstrated in Chapter 3 by Nancy Fraser, since for her gender is always already fundamentally a question of class. It is the class conflict that frames all discussions of gender, and this inevitably brackets out questions concerning rape, domestic abuse, contraception, and so on.

Today within American gender studies, the analysis of the intersection and relative independence of gender and class are always considered without question, and yet their consideration is often announced with a pretense of criticality. It is as if the American scholar of gender studies presumes that they are detracting from orthodoxy, when in actuality, they are a part of the orthodox position within their field. In this way, they become spokespersons for their field rather than interventionists. And when scholars study gender and class conflicts, there have often been discussions of 'pay equity,' 'sexual harassment' (in the workplace), 'domestic abuse,' and 'gender norms.' This is illustrated in Figure 4.1.

Queer theory eventually introduced a radically novel claim that one should focus exclusively on gender conflict in order to reveal the oppression and exploitation of language itself over the body. If classically oriented Marxists were putting forward the claim that ideology functions through key discrete institutions (such as the media, family, religious institutions, education system, and so on), then queer theorists

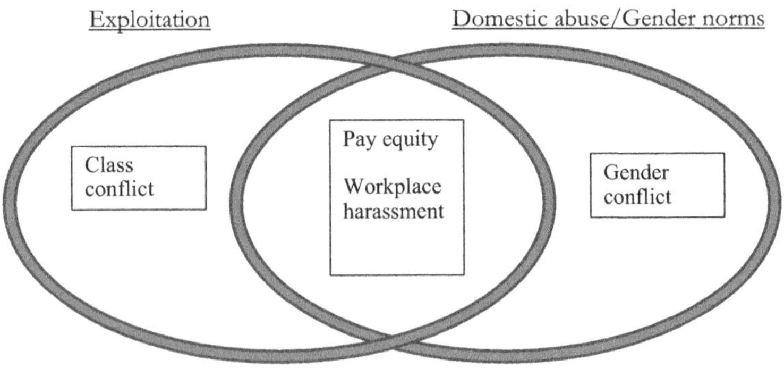

Figure 4.1 Class conflict and gender conflict

were proposing that ideology functions primarily through linguistic practices. Thus, ideology is much more pervasive among speaking beings, and it has saturated their world in a much more insidious way. Language matters. This expression – "language matters" – implies one (or both) of the following two possibilities: first, that language itself is important and that we need to understand how it functions and what role it plays in the life of human beings (i.e., we need to study language because *language* matters), and second, that language *matters*, which implies that language itself is a process of materializing the body. In the second case, we can claim that language consists of the raw materials for the construction of the reality of bodies. This is why the phrase "body of knowledge" makes sense: because a body is always made up of knowledge, and knowledge itself is always formed as a body.

We might provisionally claim that the body is real and that it is made up of 'matter.' Suppose that the biological body is real in this sense. However, queer theorists propose that language inscribes itself into or onto the biological body, substituting meaning for its stupid biology, and this is what it means to say that the body is gendered. It was for this reason that Judith Butler proposed very early a distinction between the "biological facticity" of the body and its social or linguistic "gendering" (Butler, 1988: 522). For example, she wrote that

> [W]oman is a historical idea and not a natural fact . . . [we must] underscore the distinction between sex, as biological facticity, and gender, as the cultural interpretation or signification of that facticity. To be female is, according to that distinction, a facticity which has no meaning, but to be a woman is to have become a woman, to compel the body to conform to an historical idea of 'woman,' to induce the body to become a cultural sign, to materialize oneself in obedience to an historically delimited possibility.
> (Butler, 1988: 522)

Butler here introduces the possibility that there are historical linguistic practices that dominate, tame, or otherwise simply interpret from nothing, the 'dumb' biological facticity of the body through the raw material of various historical and cultural inscriptions (ultimately, signifiers). And these cultural inscriptions are compelled to become essentialized, to posture or masquerade as 'fixed' and 'natural.' In this latter sense, signifiers are arranged by a social environment into 'signs.'

Judith Butler's theories emerged from within the general field of semiotics, a field appropriated and rearticulated by the French philosopher Jacques Derrida. Butler, a Derrida scholar who thinks within the field of gender studies, claims that the articulation of a 'sign' is always political in that it aims to conceal the differential movement of signifiers. A sign interrupts the differing and deferring of meaning at play within signification by presenting the illusion of a static and unchanging body of meaning. On the other hand, for Sigmund Freud, there is, in all actuality, something that fundamentally distinguishes the biological facticity of the body, even, and especially, within the real. We can make this claim because Freud's discourse proposes a topological twist of more naïve discourses by claiming, in his own way and perhaps without realizing it, that signifiers exist already within the real.

The so-called "narcissism of minor differences" discussed by Freud refers to the strangeness or hostility – in other words, the anxiety – produced when there are vast similarities between bodies and yet there seems to nonetheless be a minor exception. This minor exception or difference could be the genitals, and this minor difference of genitals is a form of signification from within the real itself. Yet, for many queer theorists the gendered body as a linguistic construction is absolutely to be distinguished from the inherent stupidity of the real body. Nonetheless, Butler was important for American gender studies because she helped to introduce post-structuralist assumptions into an overtly structuralist-functionalist social scientific field. Similarly, if the classical Marxist orientation was structuralist, then queer theory was decidedly 'post-structuralist.'

Structuralist Marxists presumed that there were discrete locations of power that compelled individuals to act and think in ideologically driven ways. Karl Marx and Louis Althusser each believed that the 'mode of production,' situated as the 'base,' compelled and produced the ideological superstructure. Ideas were therefore always the ideas of the dominant class, and they were used to justify, legitimize, or conceal the conflict among the bourgeoisie and proletariat occurring at the base. This was the basic model for thinking about the structure of power. Post-structuralists began with a different set of paradigmatic assumptions. One American post-structuralist has recently put it like this:

> [T]here is no center within which power is to be located. . . . There are many different sites from which it arises, and there is an interplay among these various sites in the creation of the social world. This is not to deny that there are points of concentration of power or, to keep with the spatial image, points where various (and perhaps bolder) lines intersect. [It occurs] between irreducible but mutually intersecting practices of power.
>
> (May, 1994: 11)

The post-structuralist position adopted by queer theorists may be differentiated from the preceding paradigm of the classical Marxist feminists because post-structuralism inherently presumes that power is diffuse, and consequently, that gender, in its ontological dimension, is fluid and/or radically subject to manifold symbolic interpretations. In other words, queer theory (and post-structuralist theory more broadly), displaces the mode of production from the economy onto language itself. It is not that class domination produces ideology but rather that ideology (as the conduit through which we think, the manner of manipulating language through speech, and the practice of engaging in our everyday reality) produces and reproduces various institutions and configurations of power. The primary conflict is not the economic base but rather the linguistic political-economy, which, beneath the more restrictive capitalist political-economy, gives rise to unique political-economic behaviours and institutions such as the neoliberal state.

Unlike many of the French post-structuralists, however, Judith Butler is (perhaps unknowingly) grouped among those American sociologists who are involved in the formation of a theory of 'self.' This is similar to the work of the following American sociologists: George Herbert Mead, Charles Horton Cooley, and Erving Goffman (see Rousselle, 2019). This tradition was made most popular by Herbert Blumer when he developed the phrase "symbolic interactionism" in order to group diverse American thinkers into a 'school of sociology.' For the symbolic interactionists, as well as Judith Butler, the self is socially determined. One of Butler's first major essays laid the cornerstone for the rest of her academic career: Simone de Beauvoir's claim, from *The Second Sex* (1949), that "one is not born but rather becomes woman." Based on this statement, Butler formed her theory of 'gender performativity,' developing it in the following direction:

> No biological, psychic, or economic destiny defines the figure that the human female takes on in society; it is civilization [culture] as a whole that elaborates this intermediary product between the male and the eunuch that is called feminine.
>
> (Butler, 1988)

We might derive three factors for understanding queer theory from Butler: first, there is the perspective that gender is socially determined, that is, inherited from one's social environment; second, there is the claim that gender is a product of language practices and meaning – it is a linguistic construction, which means, that it is a linguistic 'sign' that has been elevated to a culturally dominant ideological configuration; and third, there is the more obscure and often misunderstood claim that gender is a performance or an 'act.' It seems to me that this last claim retroactively weaves together the other two, since it is through the performance of gender that the subject enacts a cultural script that (s)he has inherited from the social environment. It is only through a theory of performativity that there can be something like a 'subject' who can intervene into his or her determinations. The 'script' gives direction for the performance, such that no performance can occur without a proper engagement with the script. Queer theory proposes, indeed presumes, that this script pre-exists the subject and that the subject is born into a world that compels him or her to accept the role already assigned.

Psychoanalytic theory does not find any reason to disagree with queer theory. The concept of the big 'Other' within Lacanian psychoanalytic theory describes precisely this linguistic Other, symbolic Other, which the subject internalizes in order to become an acting subject in the world. It is not true, therefore, that woman is the 'Other'

Table 4.1 The logical time of queer theory

Time 1	*Time 2*	*Time 3*
Real 'dumb' body →	Gendered inscription →	Retroactivity of the sign

sex, since that would imply that she is marked by significiations, the 'signs,' that define her among a group: *the* woman. Woman is not the Other sex precisely because Lacanians argue that she is most resistant to the Other of language and gender itself; and this is why the topic of gender is always a bit mysterious. Gender is Other in that it is the name for that practice of inscription upon the real biological facticity of the body, and femininity is precisely the name for the partial obstruction of this writing. Yet if we outline a process of logical time for queer theory, we find what is illustrated in Table 4.1.

The body pre-exists absorption by cultural signs, existing only in a 'dumb' and unintelligible reality, and then gender, as a linguistic practice, inscribes itself upon the body. Finally, through the performance of repetitive inscriptions the symbolic 'sign' stands in for the real body and retroactively naturalizes itself so that the subject can claim that "it was always this meaning, and it will always be this meaning." This script is therefore just another word for ideology, but now with the following caveat: ideology is not simply a part of the superstructure governing the fundamental conflict at the base; it is, precisely, the fundamental conflict at the base that gives rise to any super-structural harmonious political economic system.

For this reason, we can claim that ideology takes center stage within queer theory. Ideological practices are within queer theory, made up of unconscious acts that compel and determine the subject from within a social script. We find a point of agreement with Louis Althusser when he wrote that "Pascal says more or less: 'kneel down, move your lips in prayer, and you will believe.' He thus scandalously inverts the order of things . . . [and says:] language directly names reality" (Althusser, 1971). Pascal's point was that if we just practice our belief in religion or ideology then we will nonetheless believe (even if we disavow our belief). Similarly, it is through the performativity of ideology that linguistic signs gain legitimacy and help us to disavow the gender conflict. Our practices are both governed by as well as governing unconscious paradigmatic subtleties that may or may not form part of the explicit, conscious belief systems of an individual. We believe in and through our practices and performances. It does not matter if one claims to be an atheist of the religion that we name gender, what matters is that one continues to act as if one believes. We see this point made clearly in the practices of those who no longer believe in social media. Nobody today believes that Facebook, WhatsApp, Instagram, and so on are ethical forms of media, and nobody believes that we should continue to use them for our daily interactions. Yet we nonetheless continue to act as if they should form the backdrop of our daily social interactions.

Disavowal of any medium is precisely a part of the recuperative gestures of today's ideological media institutes, and they support the base of exploitation. Take another classic example from Slavoj Zizek, who wrote that "all concrete versions of this 'subject supposed to believe' (from small children for whose sake parents pretend to believe in Santa Claus, to the 'ordinary working people' for whose sake Communist intellectuals pretend to believe in Socialism) are stand-ins for the big Other" (Zizek, n.d.). He continued:

> According to a well-known anthropological anecdote, the 'primitives' to whom one attributed certain 'superstitious beliefs,' when directly asked about them, answered that 'some people believe . . . ,' immediately displacing their belief, transferring it onto another. And, again, are we not doing the same with our children: we go through the ritual of Santa Claus, since our children (are supposed to) believe in it and we do not want to disappoint them.
>
> (Zizek, n.d.)

Does this not help to explain the punchline for a popular psychoanalytic joke about a man who thought he was a piece of corn and there was a giant chicken trying to eat him? He went to his analyst and asked for a cure. After months of extensive analysis, the man was cured. Yet he returned months later and asked for help again. The psychoanalyst asks: "but I thought I cured you; you no longer believe that you are a piece of corn?" The man replies: "I know that, but the chicken doesn't know it yet!" This is how our paradigms function: at an unconscious level, at the level of the big Other, *we know very well* that our gender is assigned through citational practices within various language games, but the problem is that the Other does not know it. And it is the same for those of us who struggle within gender ideology: we know all of the politically correct gender expressions, but the chicken does not know it yet.

Citational practices within academia are often attempts to establish the legitimacy of an argument. What Judith Butler refers to as "citational practices" are similar in function to what Louis Althusser referred to as the institutes of legitimacy. Ideology has, as its chief function, the task of legitimizing conflict, to render it as a harmonious relationship, to find, within a debate, a point of agreement and rapport. Citational practices legitimize or 'essentialize' a cultural 'sign' such as 'masculinity' or 'femininity' through performative repetition. Or put differently, citational practices provide a collection of signifiers with an endurance throughout time, with a time for constancy or fixity. And the name we give to this repetition is 'sign.'

This is how gender makes the body appear as an identity. This is how gender reveals itself always as an essentialist identity. It is always through the practice of retroactively anchoring meaning to biological reality. In this sense, we can claim that gender is a not only a 'historical' phenomenon, as Judith Butler has claimed, but rather, and more precisely, we should claim that it is a 'screen memory.' For Freud, a screen memory is always an imaginary substitution of a chaotic and unpleasant reality. In this case, it is the unpleasant reality of sex. For their part, queer theorists are paradoxically anti-identitarian or anti-essentialist because they have revealed the function and fiction of language as well as the operations involved in securing this fiction we understand as the 'body.' Butler wrote: "[I]n this sense, gender is in no way a stable identity or locus of agency from which various acts proceed; rather, it is an identity tenuously constituted in time – an identity instituted through a stylized repetition of acts" (Butler, 1988: 519).

References

Ackelsberg, Martha. (1991) Free Women of Spain: Anarchism and the Struggle for the Emancipation of Women. Oakland, CA: AK Press.

Althusser, Louis. (1971) "Ideology and Ideological State Apparatuses," *Lenin and Philosophy and Other Essays* (Ben Brewster, Trans.). Monthly Review Press. As Retrieved on March 19th, 2020 from <https://www.marxists.org/reference/archive/althusser/1970/ideology.htm>

Butler, Judith. (1988) "Performative Acts and Gender Constitution: An Essay in Phenomenology and Feminist Theory," *Theatre Journal*, Vol. 40, No. 4: pp. 519–531.

May, Todd. (1994) *The Political Philosophy of Poststructuralist Anarchism*. University Park, Pennsylvania: Pennsylvania State University Press.

Rousselle, Duane. (2019) *Jacques Lacan and American Sociology: Be Wary of the Image*. London, UK: Palgrave Macmillan.

Zizek, Slavoj. (n.d.) "The Interpassive Subject," *Lacan.com*. As Retrieved on May 14th, 2019 from <www.lacan.com/interpass.htm>

5 Situating paradigms

From intersectionality to citational practices

Citational practices are ways of effortlessly repeating paradigmatic assumptions about gender. What we learn from Louis Althusser is that we are always engaged in citational practices, even and especially when we are not at all aware that we are engaged in them. It is for this reason that we can claim that it is 'unknown knowledge' rooted in the 'symbolic unconscious.' How does one get ahead in the race of the ideologues? The one who is most outside of ideology is precisely the one who admits up front that one begins in the world of gender citational practices. This is what ideology will never do: it will never begin with the presumption that it is an ideological driven creature, that the choices that seem most free are in fact already determined. On the other hand, the queer theorist is the one who has admitted to the highest degree possible within the social constructionist paradigm that citational practices exist. This, precisely, is the step that they make outside of ideology.

With Judith Butler's work in mind, we might amend Louis Althusser's statement that "there is no outside to ideology" to the following: there is no outside to gender performativity. Professors, friends, politicians, colleagues, scientists, scholars, etc. usually begin by producing the impression in us that they are not at all on the stage of ideology and that they are not involved in a performance. Too much of today's epistemological assumptions are based upon an 'evidence based' approach to truth: there is endlessly an insistence that one is free of bias, there are appeals to historical truths, and so on. These discursive manoeuvres renew the trick of ideology. Gender performativity is an ideological practice in that it includes within itself the subjective possibility of its renewal as well as its removal.

When one interrogates one's own citational practices, or when one interrogates the citational practices of the overarching social group or wider society, then one is effectively requesting to know more about one's unconscious determinations. In other words, it is a process of becoming conscious of the 'unknown knowns' that govern our gendered bodies. For example, scholars of gender within the university are typically associated with the 'social constructionist' paradigm. It too is a position that one often takes for granted, and it too demands that we repeat its fundamental presuppositions in the form of questions, declarative statements, and so on. I admit that the social constructionist paradigm has always served as a nice counterpoint to the more reductive biological or scientific essentialist paradigm.

The social constructionist paradigm reflects upon the governing presuppositions of the essentialist paradigm, and yet nonetheless, it comes also with its own foundational paradigmatic assumptions (See Table 5.1). We have been moving through some of the theories associated with each of these paradigms. These theories are meant only to serve as exemplary trends (and not as a comprehensive account of any paradigm or tradition). They serve as nodal points in the topological analyses to which I shall turn in later chapters. This accounts for the superficiality of the analyses. Classical Marxist feminist theory was later problematized by intersectional and queer theorists, though it is nonetheless situated within the same paradigm. Marxist feminisms began essentially with the assumption that gender was an issue of ideological significance, though gender may have been tied to more central and fundamental issues of social class and class conflict. Truths regarding gender were thought to be constructed at the cultural and social level (within the ideological superstructure) as a way to legitimize class conflict. Thus, we might adapt our chart in the way shown in Table 5.2.

Table 5.1 Paradigm reflexivity

	Paradigm
1	Essentialist
2	Social constructionist

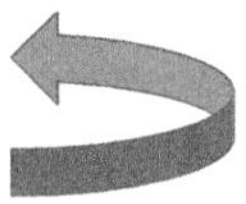

Table 5.2 Locations of the paradigm

	Paradigm	*Theory*	*Location*
1	Essentialist	Biological science	Outside university
2	Social constructionist	Marxist feminisms	Inside university
		Queer theory	→ Outside university

Judith Butler's work is perhaps the most exemplary and penultimate within the social constructionist paradigm because it seems to embody all of its assumptions in a heightened and more obvious form. The location of each theory in Table 5.2 seems to be important because today in America the confrontation is staged in the following way: the return to essentialisms, occurring largely outside of the university (and outside of the city), versus the perpetuation of social constructionist perspectives, occurring largely inside of the university but also garnering influence within the most densely populated portions of the city. And today the social constructionist perspective is under attack also by those who are within the university, those who maintain that the social constructionist perspective is a part of the ideological doctrine of the 'cultural Marxists' or the 'postmodern thinkers.' For example, see this statement made by Jordan Peterson:

> There is no limit to what ideologues are going to sacrifice to their ideology, and that obviously includes children. . . . That whole idea of intersectionality is one of the weakest intellectual ideas I've ever encountered. One of the strange things about these ideas that have become current – the idea of white privilege, the idea of the patriarchy, the idea of intersectionality, the idea of safe spaces and toxic masculinity, and trigger warnings, and micro-aggressions – is that they are developed by sociological thinkers with no empirical evidence whatsoever and with absolutely no knowledge whatsoever of how to do proper measure, and no notion that there is even a science that knows how to do that . . . much less knowing anything about biology.
>
> (Peterson, 2018)

What we notice from Peterson's explanation is that he is anchored to the essentialist paradigm, but in a way that is in communication with (and not at all in ignorance of) the social constructionist set of assumptions. On a few points, nonetheless, Peterson is correct: we do not typically see essentialist discourses within sociology and gender studies departments. In fact, as sociologists or gender studies scholars we typically only ever mention essentialist assumptions so that we can critique them.

'Essentialist' is almost exclusively reserved as one of the 'bad words' of sociology, and it signifies not only an attack on a set of assumptions, but by implication, an attack upon assumptions that make up the common opinions for Americans. Therefore, to understand essentialist assumptions we also are required to understand social constructionist assumptions: the social constructionists were among those who discovered and analyzed essentialist assumptions. For example, it was the discovery of the social constructionists to mark a distinction between 'sex' and 'gender.' Already we saw how this distinction was drawn by Judith Butler within her discussion of the 'biological facticity' of sex (or the body) and 'gender' as a citational practice. Whereas gender involves the symbolic domain (e.g., meanings, language, scripts, interpretation, and so on), sex involves the 'dumb' reality of the body.

One of the fundamental moves made by the Judith Butler and the queer theorists – this was a move also made by many other theorists within the social constructionist paradigm – was to insist upon the distinction between sex and gender. It was a subtle but forceful attack upon the essentialist conviction that sex and gender are synonymous. Today the essentialist paradigm is resurrected in America by President Donald Trump, who, like the University of Toronto professor Jordan Peterson, appeals to populist reasoning by claiming that the perspective of the two, that is, the perspective that insists upon two words ('sex' and 'gender'), is superfluous. Thus, there is no requirement for two words: one word suffices; gender is 'sex.'

We might claim that the conflation of sex and gender necessitates a movement into ideology. However, on the other hand, the perspective of the 'one,' the perspective of the social constructionists, is *a priori* ideological: all the more because the claim is that there is an unchanging truth or biological facticity about the body that nonetheless unknowingly comes only through the assurances of language (e.g., birth certificate, medical documents, etc.). This is shown also in the case of Donald Trump (see Green et al., 2018). When we make epistemological claims, truth claims, about the body we are in effect claiming without argument what we consciously know while retreating from any examination of the 'unknown knowns' of the body. We exchange reflexivity for naïve certainty.

The critical gesture of social constructionism was to have unearthed the 'unknown knowns' of the body that are already existing at the foundation of our essentialist narratives. It was only by producing a 'cut' – an epistemic distinction between sex and gender – that the 'other scene' of gender as ideology became exposed. It is only in this sense that we may suggest that the social constructionists are reflexive, in that they are reflexive essentialists. The social constructionists are at their worst when they charge others with essentialism, thereby posturing at freeing themselves from the script that nonetheless determines them. Conversely, the social constructionists are at their best when they affirm wholeheartedly that they are in fact determined by the script of gender, and that consequently, it is by admitting this up front that they stand a chance of stepping outside of the performance.

The position that claims (if only implicitly) that gender *is* sex also claims without realizing it that the unconscious is completely made conscious. It amounts to statements similar to the following: "I am always completely conscious of myself," "I am entirely self-aware," "I am the master of my fate," "I think therefore I am," and so on. Thus, the essentialist position is always the one that denigrates and rejects the unconscious. The essentialist subject will always be in denial of ideology, of the fact of unconscious determinations, and so on. It is in this way that their denial of the unconscious only subjects them all the more to its various determinations. It is by producing the 'cut' that separates sex from gender, the cut which extracts out of sex the discovery of gender, that we can begin to assert that there exists a dimension of the 'unknown knowns' and that there are meanings that we take for granted.

The social constructionist paradigm therefore begins with the presumption that gender is ideological, that it is a cultural or social configuration inherited from the social environment by the subject. We are always in the 'prison-house' of gender. Gender imprisons the real sexed body through cultural significations. On the other hand, sex, in its real facticity outside of language, is a profound site of contestation: there are gender wars involved in citational practices, and from within the social environment there are various tendencies that try to colonize the body and to pass itself off as its final truth. To cause "gender trouble," as Butler puts it, then, is not at all to resist the script. This is not the point, since this only reproduces the problem. On the contrary, we have to be careful: by wilfully stepping outside of the script of gender we renew the trick of ideology. Instead, the critical gesture is to 'denaturalize sex,' or 'to uncouple sex from itself,' in order to expose the split that already exists within the culture of the body. We might summarize all of this in a simple way, as shown in Table 5.3.

The perspective of the 'one' is defined by the presumption that gender is equal to sex, while the perspective of the 'two' presumes that gender is not equal to sex. I use traditional Boolean symbols "!=" to denote "not equal to," and the double "==" to indicate "equal to." I have placed "*" beside the theory of intersectionality because it is a new theory, and I want to demonstrate that it is situated within the perspective of the two.

In many ways, bell hooks problematized the classical Marxist feminist theoretical orientation. Against the reductive position of the 'two,' which placed class conflict at the center of all analyses, intersectional theory has positioned the various zones of conflict within

Table 5.3 Two perspectives

Perspective	*Paradigm*	*Theory*
One (Gender == sex)	Essentialist	Trumpism
Two (Gender != sex)	Social constructionist	Marxist feminism (Nancy Fraser) *Intersectionality (bell hooks) Queer theory (Judith Butler)

an overall 'matrix of domination.' Incidentally, bell hooks discovered first hand at an early age the power of language. Indeed, she was born "Gloria Jean Watkins" but changed her name to bell hooks, all lower case, as a sign of humility. This no doubt marks an attempt to interrupt the patriarchal citational practices of Western societies, but it also opens up an interesting question about the American fascination with self-nomination.

For example, there is an optional practice of self-nomination at Grand Valley State University, in Allendale, Michigan, United States. At the institutional level there is a new policy titled "MyName," which permits students to remove a lot of the pressures associated with the gendered ideological citational practices of our names. On the university website, the following is written: "[a]t Grand Valley State University, we recognize that an individual may wish to be identified by a professional, personal, preferred, display or use a name without making an official legal name change" (GVSU, 2019). On the whole, as faculty and students, we tend to accept this as a progressive move on the part of the institution. However, as a professor I am able to see a reality hidden from the students. The institution has only produced an 'overlay' system such that the preferred name only *appears* to replace the legal name while the underlying reality remains nonetheless the same. The preferred name is placed onto the online classroom software, onto class lists, and even onto degrees; nonetheless, the student's legal name remains in the background on all of the files securing the preferred name: the institution is nonetheless anchored to state and federal practices regarding birth certificates, Social Security numbers, and so on. It is only at the surface, in the imaginary, at the level of appearances, that there has been a change. As such, it only *appears* to solve the problem of gender discrimination while renewing it as a more insidious problem through its obscuration.

It is even possible that the overlay system produces an appearance of linguistic gender harmony without exposing the fundamental problem that remains at the core of the government citational practice: it therefore only renews the ideological trap. Rather than to directly confront the conflict at the level of the government – official documents and student records which remain secretly anchored to government citational practices – students are now superficially satisfied, and there is a return to the essentialist paradigm rather than an attack upon it through its exposition. Professors, for their part, are compelled to ignore (through several private emails with instructions to professors about how to cite the overlay system rather than the official records system) the base system of official documents.

hooks draws from her personal biography to discuss her experiences at the intersection of poverty and racism during an early age. On the one hand, racism is experienced in of itself, and yet capitalist exploitation also exacerbates those problems. Indeed, one of hooks' earliest experiences was of 'talking back' to her teachers and classmates. This is an expression I quite like because it indicates a turn back to the social script that surrounds her; it is a topological twist, if I may put it like that, or rather, a reflexive questioning of the declarative statements of the social script on race, gender, and class. The dominant voice at that time was 'white,' 'male,' and 'middle class.' To 'talk back' to the dominant voice was to assert a subjective position within white-capitalist-patriarchy (hooks, 1989).

'Talking back' implies for hooks that she no longer wanted to imitate or repeat the citational practices of white middle-class women. She thereby exposed the inadequacy of those citational practices by demonstrating that there was an ingrained exclusion of the experiences and voices of poor black women. Indeed, hooks, as a young adult, began to experiment with the malleability of language itself. She turned to poetry. Whereas philosophers and psychoanalysts (since at least the time of Martin Heidegger and Jacques Lacan) have claimed that language tortures the subject – Heidegger used to refer to the "prison-house of language" – Zizek, through Elfriede Jelinek, claims that "language [itself] should be tortured [back] to tell the truth" (Zizek, 2014: 871). He continues to say that "it should be twisted, denaturalized, extended, condensed, cut, and reunited, made to work against itself. . . . The most elementary form of torturing one's language is called poetry" (Zizek, 2014). We should nonetheless be very careful: the social constructionists were correct in claiming that linguistic practices determine our gender, yet constructionism is at its worst when it begins to claim that we may just construct the world however we like through our self-conscious language practices.

This latter problematic belief has opened up a zone of conscious language practices that have brought us down the dark pathway of political correctness. Although language determines us, it does not follow that we are somehow able to so easily determine language. The essentialist contribution of queer theory is not that we may construct and create our meanings and identities however we please. As we shall see, that only returns us to and renews the fundamental problem of erasing the unconscious. It is a much more radical position than social constructionism: any such attempt is doomed to fall back into the confines of ideology. In any case, the 'prison-house of language' is at no time more apparent than when an individual falls in love with another person. For the person in love, each word is like a prison-bar trapping the subject inside the inadequacy of language: "words cannot express what I feel for you!"

There is here nonetheless something 'queer' about poetry because the poet discovers the 'prison-house of language' and yet instead of feeling tortured decides instead to be the one who tortures: and the manner in which one tortures is to reveal, through language, the citational practices themselves: "Ain't I a Woman?" At the age of 19, hooks wrote her first major book, titled *Ain't I a Woman: Black Women and Feminism* (1981). The title of her book was an obvious reference to a speech made by the African American slavery abolitionist Sojourner Truth, a speech that many scholars have identified as among the first of the American 'intersectional' positions. The book interrogated the pretense of exclusivity for those who deploy the epistemological category of 'woman.' 'Woman' was for them a category claiming universal representability, yet it did not at all include the unique perspectives of conflict experienced by those outside of middle class or Caucasian women. If it is true, as Simone de Beauvoir claimed, that "one is not born a woman but becomes one," then it would seem that even *that* dignity had not been granted to black women.

Another way that hooks has tortured language was by discussing "feminist movement" rather than "*the* feminist movement." The difference was in the removal of the definite article, "the," which, when written endlessly within her texts, disrupted the sense in which feminist movement consists of a monolithic group organized around an apparent (but ever exclusive) shared identity. When you use the definite article, you also presume that the reader already has some knowledge about the referent: it is a *supposed* knowledge. For this reason, the definite article is always an ingredient within ideological thought because it introduces a citational practice of the formation of supposed body of knowledge essentialized through the logic of identity. bell hooks aimed to disrupt this tendency of essentializing by demonstrating through her own citational practices that feminism or feminist movement is not the same for everybody. Indeed, there are different situated knowledges and perspectives, different situated experiences and identities, different experiences of conflict and power/privilege, and so on.

Similar approaches were developed by the American sociologist Patricia Hill Collins. For example, in *Black Feminist Thought: Knowledge, Consciousness and the Politics of Empowerment* (1990), Collins, a former president of the American Sociological Association, began to focus on the intersection of race and gender, but also on those unique experiences of black women within academia. This latter debate occurred in her article from *Social Problems* in 1986, titled "Learning From the Outsider Within: The Sociological Significance of Black Feminist Thought." She wrote:

> Black women have long occupied marginal positions in academic settings. I argue that many Black female intellectuals have made creative use of their marginality – their 'outsider within' status, to produce Black feminist thought that reflects the standpoint on self, family, and society.
>
> (Collins, 1986: 14)

Here, we can see the importance of 'standpoint,' of the various differently constituted identities and practices, for the formation of paradigmatic behaviours and thoughts. It was this position that led her to discuss the interlocking nature of oppression. I shall quote it at length:

> The Black feminist attention to the interlocking nature of oppression is significant. . . . First, this viewpoint shifts the entire focus of investigation from one aimed at explicating the elements of race or gender or class oppression to one whose goal is to determine what the links are among these systems. The first approach typically prioritizes one form of oppression as being primary, then handles remaining types of oppression as variables within what is seen as the most important system. For example, the efforts to insert race and gender into Marxist theory exemplify this effort. In contrast, the more holistic approach implied in Black feminist thought treats the interaction among multiple systems as the object of study.
>
> (Collins, 1990: 20)

It seems to me that this is among the most precise definitions for the approach today referred to as 'intersectionality' inside of the university, but also outside of it within activist communities. The challenge for hooks was to think of feminist movement as composed of diverse perspectives, multiple sites of struggle, and multiple identities (e.g., gender, race, class).

Although Kimberle Crenshaw, an American scholar and lawyer, first used the concept of intersectionality in 1989, hooks nonetheless demonstrated the same conceptual approach in her usage of the phrase "imperialist-supremacist-capitalist-patriarchy" in *Feminist Theory: From Margin to Center* (1984). To summarize this point: intersectionality implies, minimally, that there is not only an interlocking system of domination within the social structure but also that there are, consequently, distinct situated experiences, identities, and knowledges. The goal is to disrupt any tendency that aims at the fixation of any particular identity (such as the 'proletariat'). Relatedly, the aim is to disrupt the ingrained tendency among activist and progressive (for lack of a better word) scholars to focus only upon one axis of power such as capitalist exploitation.

However, the problem is also that people do not quite know what intersectionality is. Is it a concept or an orientation or a theory? Some have even claimed that it is a buzzword (Davis, 2008). Kathy Davis wrote: “[we] are all convinced that intersectionality is [now] absolutely essential to feminist theory . . . but we are not at all sure what the concept means” (Davis, 2008). Minimally, we can claim that intersectionality brings the concept of identity to the fore precisely by pluralizing the concept as ‘identities.’ The concept of intersectionality certainly became increasingly popular within gender studies departments and sociology departments in the last few decades. Davis wrote: “[a]t this particular juncture in gender studies, any scholar who neglects difference runs the risk of having her work viewed as theoretically misguided, politically, irrelevant, or simply fantastical” (Davis, 2008: 68). Intersectionality has provided an intensified focus on the differential quality of identities.

Queer theory, in a different way, has also contributed to this heightened emphasis on the differential quality of identities. If intersectionality mapped situated but discrete differences, then queer theory demonstrated that even within the overarching category of gender there are differences all the way down. I shall turn now to this topic in the next chapter.

References

Collins, Patricia. (1986) “Learning from the Outsider within: The Sociological Significance of Black Feminist Thought,” *Social Problems*, Vol. 33, No. 6: pp. 14–32.

Davis, Kathy. (2008) “Intersectionality as Buzzword: A Sociology of Science Perspective on What Makes a Feminist Theory Successful,” *Feminist Theory*, Vol. 9, No. 1: pp. 67–85.

Green, Erica L., Benner, Katie, & Pear, Robert. (2018) “‘Transgender Could Be Defined Out of Existence under Trump Administration,” *New York Times*, October 21. As Retrieved on May 31st, 2019 from <www.nytimes.com/2018/10/21/us/politics/transgender-trump-administration-sex-definition.html>

GVSU. (2019) “MyName,” As Retrieved on May 31st, 2019 from <www.gvsu.edu/myname/>

hooks, bell. (1981) *Ain't I a Woman: Black Women and Feminism*. Boston, MA: South End Press.

hooks, bell. (1984) *Feminist Theory: From Margin to Center*. Abingdon, UK: Routledge.

hooks, bell. (1989) *Talking Back: Thinking Feminist, Thinking Black*. Toronto, Canada: Between the Lines Press.

Patricia Hill Collins. (1990) Black Feminist Thought: Knowledge, Consciousness and the Politics of Empowerment, Australia: Unwin Hyman.

Peterson, Jordan. (2018) "Jordan Peterson: Intersectionality Theory Is Weak," [Video] As Retrieved on May 15th, 2019 from <www.youtube.com/watch?v=69cLbhf6jV8>

Zizek, Slavoj. (2014) "The Poetic Torture-House of Language," *Poetry*. As Retrieved on May 17th, 2019 from <www.poetryfoundation.org/poetrymagazine/articles/70096/the-poetic-torture-house-of-language>

6 Interrogating intersectionality

Joya Misra has written a wonderful chapter in *Gender Reckonings* (2018) addressing the "theory war" occurring during the last few decades between intersectional theorists and queer theorists. The latter, queer theory, is referred to more broadly as 'post-structuralist theory.' However, to keep things simple, we might claim that 'queer theory' is the name for post-structuralist theory when it occurs within the more restrictive field of gender studies. Misra is of the opinion that the intersectional approach is the one to which we ought to hold onto and give primacy, but only after thoroughly engaging with the challenges posed by queer theory. For my part, I do not want to rush to judgment. Rather, I would like to begin to map or chart these theories so that we might understand how they are situated in relation to one another. This approach avoids the normative judgments of the perspective of the 'one.'

Our simple chart has hitherto plotted a few paradigms and some respective theories without taking into account some of the foundational concepts associated with each of the respective theories. It seems to me that there is no better existing concept that is capable of expressing what is most singular about intersectional theory than the following one from Patricia Hill Collins: "matrix of domination" Collins, Patricia (1990). This is a more advanced explanation for understanding the source of domination since a matrix is by definition the environment within which something develops. The matrix of domination describes the environment of domination, in all its various registers. It implies that the social environment is complex and fragmented. Each subject is uniquely situated within that matrix and this produces relative advantages and disadvantages, privileges and oppressions, etc.

The matrix of domination configures our various identities in unique and subtle ways, such that a universal and essential identity that expresses our shared experiences of suffering within the social environment can no longer be presumed. It is always possible that we suffer and dominate each other in unique ways depending on our relative situatedness within the matrix. It is for this reason that intersectionality typically welcomes any theory of situated knowledges, since to be situated in this case means to be placed differently within the environment. Consider the relationship of this theory to that of Georg Lukacs in his *History & Class Consciousness* (1923):

> [T]he knowledge yielded by the standpoint of the proletariat stands on a higher scientific plane objectively; it does after all apply a method that makes possible the solution of problems which the greatest thinkers of the bourgeois era have vainly struggled to find and in its substance, it provides the adequate historical analysis of capitalism which must remain beyond the grasp of bourgeois thinkers.

It is from a particular vantage point that one class approaches a higher scientific plane, or in other words, epistemological objectivity. This occurs precisely because of one's location within the capitalist structure of domination. Within feminist theory, the equivalent was 'feminist standpoint theory,' which becomes more nuanced as it approaches intersectional situated theories.

This overall position concerning the situated dimension of truth was developed in a rather interesting way in recent years by Slavoj Zizek wrote:

> [A] parallax view [is a] constantly shifting perspective between two points between which no synthesis or mediation is possible. Thus, there is no rapport between the two levels, no shared space – although they are closely connected, even identical in a way, they are, as it were, on the opposed sides of a Mobius strip.
>
> *The Parallax View* (2009: 4)

In a restrictive sense, a parallax view describes the situated perspectives of the proletariat and the bourgeoisie within the domain of ideology. Although they begin from fundamentally different points of departure (e.g., the one beginning with M1 and the other with C1), they nonetheless both occur on the same basic surface. As Marxists, we name this 'surface' bourgeois ideology, since all ideology is the ideology of the ruling class. What, then, of ideology within the perspective of intersectional and queer theories? We cannot claim that ideology ceases to function – rather it becomes more insidious because it relies increasingly upon citational practices.

Increasingly, we discuss not 'standpoint,' but *standpoints* (plural). We have progressed by pluralizing *the* word. We now discuss the movement of 'movements,' identity becomes 'identities,' standpoint becomes 'standpoints'; now, we see also, with Donna Haraway (1988), that situated knowledge becomes 'situated knowledges.' Yet, even here, Haraway is focused on internal differences within a given gender category: feminist objectivity and empiricism, like proletarian knowledge, is different from masculine scientific objectivity or bourgeois knowledge. The problem was that Haraway, and others, could not see that what makes this difference is precisely the parallax gap of reflexivity and acceptance of one's situatedness within ideology.

These concepts – matrix of domination, situated knowledges, standpoints, and so on – are themselves situated within the social constructionist paradigm. In every case, we are presuming that the subject suffers within a social environment, and that consequently, there are different epistemological assumptions related to the location from which a subject speaks or writes. Unlike the essentialist paradigm and its various theories, social constructionists assume that we always situate subjects with various social determinants. The essentialist perspective begins rather with the outlook that we are all biologically determined. This distinction has become of such importance that I now would like to discuss them in terms of the perspective of the 'one' and the perspective of the 'two.'

I situate 'intersectionality' and 'queer theory' within the perspective of the 'two,' the social constructionist paradigm. Both positions share the same paradigmatic assumption. It does not matter if we use the conceptual vocabulary of the 'matrix of domination' or the 'performativity of gender' because in both cases we are tied to the same paradigmatic assumption that gender is determined or inherited by the social environment. Nonetheless, within the social constructionist paradigm there are modes of distinguishing the various theories, whether they be Marxist feminist, intersectional, or queer. For example, we might use the variables of 'identity' and 'universalism' to outline a subtle distinction between intersectionality and queer theory. At first sight, these two concepts seem to be tied to the essentialist perspective; however, the difference is that within the essentialist paradigm we can expect an uncritical acceptance of identity without the associated reflexive nomination implied through linguistic practices. On the other hand, the social constructionist paradigm exposes, names, and critically interrogates the concepts of identity and universality.

Essentialists take for granted the fact of identity, allowing it to form the content of their 'unknown knowledge' of gender, and they do so, also often without realizing it, to elevate their discourse to the universal position. They will claim that the biological determinations of the body, as certified by government documents, are true for all cases. On the other hand, the social constructionists attempt to work themselves out of this position by proclaiming themselves to be subjected to the matrices of domination and their various citational practices. Or, put another way, they work themselves out of gender ideology by paradoxically proclaiming themselves to be determined by operative identities that strive for epistemological universality.

The essentialist paradigm begins with the assumption that there is something unchanging, natural, and necessary concerning our gender identity. For example, the claim that "all men have penises," or "all men have XY chromosomes," is intended to be universally binding. It relies on the assumptions of biological science, and it disavows the linguistic citational portion that nonetheless legitimizes it "as certified by government documents." It is therefore a mathematical statement: "For all *xy*, it is true that . . ." This is the source of universalist logic for the essentialists. Put another way, the essentialist paradigm presumes that sex is equal to gender, and that therefore, gender is not a term worth deploying. The basic assumption is that only one word is required: *sex*. This is what defines the perspective of the 'one.' It is the universality of the one gender, which, for adherents of the paradigm, is not assigned but is rather declared, and is universally true. It is an epistemological universality without any acceptance of the fact of its own point of exception within language.

Identity is more operative within the essentialist paradigm, but it is the social constructionist paradigm that claims responsibility for this discovery. An identity fixes meaning, secures it in place. Its English variant indicates, since the 1600s, 'sameness' or 'oneness.' From the Medieval Latin word *idem*, which means 'same,' it also carries a sense of being 'the same as before,' or rather, 'the same *one* as before.' The social constructionist discovers, within the essentialist perspective, that identity is secured through the citational practices of that which is currently 'the same as before,' which means that it is a mere repetition. It is from within this citational practice, which implies that the 'one' becomes removed from itself and made into 'two.' Identity is secured by proclaiming that something came before and that it was therefore secured through a repetition. Sex is therefore equal to gender because of a citational practice.

Trumpian discourse secures an ostensibly natural gender identity for the subject by claiming that our gender is "the same as it was before," the same as it was when we were born. This, at least, was the claim put forth in Trump's leaked memo as revealed on October 21st, 2018, in the *New York Times* (Green et al., 2018). Trump was involved without knowing it in the attempt to 'make gender great *again*,' and yet he can only appeal to the past, by therefore repeating it, in order to secure his universally binding doctrine. Moreover, he is forced to produce for himself a linguistic sign that would take on a cultural signification: one refers only to the certification of the government document, via the birth certificate. It is only from within the social constructionist paradigm that we can better understand the essentialist paradigm. It is the defining feature of social constructionism to diagnose the problems of identity and universality within the essentialist paradigm.

The social constructionist paradigm produces a new situated knowledge precisely by discovering social and linguistic determinations within the preceding essentialist paradigm. Put psychoanalytically, these determinations are of the 'big Other,' since the big Other is responsible for installing our desires via the conduit of language and the social environment. Desire is always the desire of the big Other.

Through this discovery, the perspective of the two demonstrates to us that Trump's discourse is not only essentialist but also politically reactionary. To be reactionary implies that one returns to the comforts of the existing state of affairs. The reactionary subject is the one who is confronted with the reality of anxiety and uncertainty by recoiling, retreating, reacting by returning to the way things have already been or the way things already were: to make gender great *again*. Although it seems as though the essentialist paradigm is reactionary at its core, it is not clear that it in fact is. Yet within academia, it is as if the only role for the perspective of the two is to reveal the reactionary core of essentialist gender politics.

Moreover, it is only by beginning with the perspective of the two that we might begin to admit that there is such a thing as ideology, and that we are always already situated within the structure of ideology. Although it is not necessary for us to admit that we are all situated uniquely within ideology, it is nonetheless necessary for us to admit that there is some existence of ideology – this is the minimum condition to be involved in the unique vantage points of the second perspective. This, I believe, is its most essential contribution to gender studies. Incidentally, it is only from within the social constructionist paradigm that we can begin to discuss the essentialist paradigm. This is because the essentialist perspective does not see itself as a perspective at all. The oddity is that the essentialist perspective pre-exists its own awareness and diagnosis. The essentialist paradigm existed before the social constructionist, but we would not have known it without the reflexivity of the perspective of the two. There can be no discovery of the logic of the one without a vantage point from within the logic of the two.

So two precedes one, logically. Does the perspective of the two not cut the perspective of the one, exposing this cut as already being operative anyway? If, within the essentialist perspective, *sex is not equal to gender* (and so there is one word required), then within the perspective of the two, for the first time, the distinction between sex and gender – the insistence upon there being two words to make sense of one, sex – occurs. The perspective of the two does not posit that *sex == gender*, but rather that *sex != gender*, which means, in other words, that sex is never entirely reducible to gender (and vice versa).

It is by exposing the cut within gender, by writing, as I do, *sex != gender*, that we challenge the universalist pretensions of essentialist gender identity formations. It is not that the concept and problem of identity disappears for the perspective of the two but rather that we discover that there is nothing natural or essential about gender identity at all: sex is a site of profound contestation, and it is not at all fixed *for all*.

It is from within this perspective also that we realize that the *for all* of universalist identity always comes with an inherent exclusion: there will always be another situated knowledge, another identity that has not yet been accounted from within the matrixial configuration of our own sociological scripts. In other words, when it comes to sex, we can never 'say it all.' Epistemology fails in matters concerning sexuality, and yet paradoxically, it is the failure of sex that is also the mark of its success: we can never say it all about sex, and this is why, nonetheless, we can always say something else about sex. Within the category of the proletariat, there was an exclusion of the feminine; within the category of the feminine, there was an exclusion of race, and class, and so on. We discover therefore that gender is not only distinguished from sex but that through this distinction gender experiences a paradoxical limitation: it is an epistemology always up against a limit, it is an epistemology limited by the real unknowability of sex itself.

I have until now introduced a few key words shared by the two major paradigms or perspectives: 'identity,' 'language,' 'universalism.' Once again, the universal position is often thought to mean that *for all x* (or, rather, for all *XY* or *XX*) there is something essential and true. It is an epistemological universalism. In this way, epistemological universalism always engages the unconscious, even when it occurs outside of Trumpian discourse in the first wave of the feminist movement. Indeed, the first wave secured its universalist pretensions (e.g., to represent *all women;* "for all women . . .") without acknowledging its inherent exclusion: poor African American women, and numerous other unacknowledged identities. This was what the intersectional theorists discovered, many of whom were among the excluded 'non-part' striving for inclusion. For example, there is the claim that *for all women, it is true that pay equity is the pressing issue*. It is only through our entrance to the perspective of the two that we open up an awareness to the logic of the exception.

Therefore, it is not true that gender essentialism is something that only other people are tied to. It occurred within the more progressive first wave feminist movement while it also occurred recently in the more regressive or reactionary Trumpian discourse. Indeed, gender essentialisms exist across the various political spectrums, and also within sociology and gender studies departments. There are reactionary and progressive essentialisms. The progressive essentialisms were those of the first wave, whose concerns were for pay equity, the right to vote, and the right to enter into public discourse or the public sphere. When we claim that a discourse is 'progressive,' we mean to suggest that it attempted to produce a 'cut,' which forces an interrogation of unfair power and resource distributions with society. There is here an attempt to form a 'two,' but only by externalizing the two throughout society: men and women, the proletariat and the bourgeoisie, and so on.

The progressive position is always the one that confronts the possibility of a thinking that counts, a thinking of the two. How it cuts the two matters very little, for our purposes; in essentialist progressivisms the two becomes externalized onto society itself, since society itself becomes cut by gender. The two of gender is cut out from the one of sex. The reactionary position occurs when there is the exposition of a two, which frightens the subject into stitching it back together into a one. This is precisely the orientation of Trumpian discourse when it confronts the possibility of transgender: the two must be sutured into one, the differences must be overcome in favour once again of the renewal of a universality without exception. We must make gender great again. Reactionary politics is always a politics that cannot and will not count. Moreover, what was once progressive, such as the first wave of *the* feminist movement, can later become critiqued as reactionary; and what was once reactionary can in turn become reactivated as progressive. Here, I mean only to set the stage for the chapters which follow.

In the simplified chart in Table 6.1, the left column indicates that the concept of identity is present but not consciously admitted within the perspective of the one. It is consciously admitted and hence it is

Table 6.1 The simplified chart

(+) Identity				*(-) Language*
	Paradigm	*Theory*	*Concept*	
	Essentialist	Trumpism	Biology/gov. certification	
		1st wave feminism	Pay equity Right to vote	
	Social construct-ionist	Classical Marxist feminism	Exploitation Surplus value ideology	
		inter-sectionality	Matrix of domination Situated knowledges Performativity	
		Queer theory	Citational practices	
(-) Identity				(+) Language

paradoxically less present within the perspective of the two. The right column indicates that language is not thought to be important in the first perspective, while it becomes of increasing significance within the later theories of the second perspective. It is through language (e.g., the raw materials which the subject inherits from the social environment) that something like identity is possible at all. Thus, there is a reflexive twist included within the second perspective, and this reflexive twist demonstrates the intimate connection of language and the social environment to the unconscious.

References

Collins, Patricia. (1990) *Black Feminist Thought: Knowledge, Consciousness, and the Politics of Empowerment*. Boston: Unwin Hyman.

Green, Erica, Benner, Katie, & Pear, Robert. (2018) "'Transgender' Could Be Defined Out of Existence under Trump Administration," *The New York Times*, October 21. As Retrieved on May 22nd, 2019 from <www.nytimes.

com/2018/10/21/us/politics/transgender-trump-administration-sex-definition.html>

Haraway, Donna. (1988) "Situated Knowledges: The Science Question in Feminism and the Privilege of Partial Perspective," *Feminist Studies*, Vol. 14, No. 3: pp. 575–599.

Lukacs, Georg. (1923) "The Standpoint of the Proletariat," in *History & Class Consciousness*. As Retrieved on May 22nd, 2019 from <www.marxists.org/archive/lukacs/works/history/hcc07_1.htm>

Misra, Joya. (2018) "Categories, Structures, and Intersectional Theory," in *Gender Reckonings: New Social Theory and Research* (James W. Messerschmidt, Michael A. Messner, Raewyn Connell, & Patricia Martin, Eds.). New York: New York University Press. pp. 111–129.

Zizek, Slavoj. (2009) *The Parallax View*. Cambridge, MA: MIT Press.

7 Psychoanalysis and gender

The Mobius strip

The essentialist paradigm has a universalist conviction with respect to gender identity, with only a minor awareness of the possibility of any exception. The social constructionist paradigm, on the other hand, presumes that there is an exception – in order to displace, challenge, and prefigure the concept of identity. In this case, an exception is understood as that which not only resists universalist epistemological inscriptions but also that which insists upon its renewal. The exception is that which resists universal inscription and yet it is also that which insists upon being inscribed or included within the universal framework. It is that which gives rise to the critique of identity (as demonstrated by the theories of intersectionality and in some forms of Marxist feminisms), but it is also that which gives rise to the *affirmation* of new identities (as demonstrated by the concept of 'genderfluid' and in the proliferation of situated identities).

Gender is not simply (or only) responsible for inscribing itself upon the real sexed body, although this seems to be the central claim made from within the social constructionist perspective. Sex is also responsible for interrupting any of the social scripts that we inherit. The sexed body is not only a surface upon which the language of the big Other or social environment is written, it is also the point at which language breaks down and becomes reformulated. Therefore, we have had three points of departure, or three paradigms: essentialist, social constructionist, and also a new third perspective or paradigm that introduces what was previously unacknowledged but operative within the truth procedure of the second. The perspective of the 'three' discovers what has not yet been acknowledged as its principal truth within the perspective of the 'two': the real of 'sex.'

There is a biological facticity to the sexed body, and this is why we can claim that sex exists independent of our thinking and interpreting it. This biological facticity certainly exists outside of the interpretations inherited from society. The essentialist perspective names this 'sex.' But there is also the social construction of the sexed body: the body becomes coded with meanings, and finally, fixed into a cultural sign. We name this practice 'gender' or 'ideology.' Finally, there is now a question concerning the relationship of 'sex' and 'gender': gender writes upon the sexed body but it will always confront a zone that cannot be coded. There will always be something *more to say* about the body, there will always be another identity, another possible citational practice, and so on. And the reason for possibility of always saying more is the following: there is something *real* about the sexed body that absolutely resists symbolization.

This is why we can claim that the social constructionist paradigm is not necessarily universalist. There is always an exception. The social constructionist paradigm exposes the exception of the sexed body itself. We have moved therefore from the discovery of the 'symbolic unconscious' of the body, an ideological body coded with 'unknown knowledges,' toward the third perspective, the 'real unconscious,' or a real sexed body. We are not therefore anymore in the perspective of the 'one' because we realize that there are indeed infinite identities available to us. But we are also no longer within the perspective of the 'two' because we are no longer interested only in suggesting that identities are inherited and that there are still ever more symbolic identities that are yet to be discovered. Indeed, we must be careful of the perspective of the 'multiple' – which elaborates a theory of mutliplicitous identities and registers of power or conflict – because this is a deceitful position. Any position that presumes that there are an infinite supply of gender or identity configurations, and then it sometimes goes on at length to archive and categorize them, is a part of the perspective of the 'multiple.'

Such a progressive position runs the risk of transforming into a reactionary position. The one attempts to have the last word on gender. However, at times the two also attempts to have the last word on gender by exposing a zone of conflict between sex and gender. In this way, the two is certainly an attack upon any one. However, the 'multiple,' as a possibility within the 'two,' attempts to pass itself off as a two when in fact it regresses into the affirmation of a multiplicity of ones as its rejection of identity. The 'multiple' is an attempt to have the last word on gender by suggesting one of the following:

1 Gender is not anymore ideology or ideologically determined for the subject, and that therefore, there are no longer any scripts to which the subject is forced to cite, and/or that the subject is now fully conscious and able to step outside of its ideological determinations; and/or
2 We can capture and understand all of the various identity configurations within the matrix of domination, and therefore say it all about the sexed body.

When we take the position of the 'multiple,' we have therefore only regressed to the perspective of the 'one' by proclaiming ourselves no longer dupes of ideology. This is how the "non-dupes err" (to borrow an expression from Jacques Lacan) within the social constructionist perspective. In his seminar of November 13th, 1973, Lacan said that "the unconscious is indeed the support of . . . a knowledge. . . . [T]he non-dupes who err means that anyone who is not in love with his unconscious errs" (Lacan, 1973: 20). At the very least, to be in love with the unconscious is to begin from the perspective of the 'two,' but it is not to remain there, and it is not to become the 'non-dupes' of the one: the penultimate achievement of the social constructionist paradigm was to proclaim that one is in fact a dupe of one's unconscious. The challenge is to remain committed to this progressive impulse of the social constructionist paradigm and not to be tempted by the reactionary potential of the multiple.

We should, for example, locate the progressive orientation within the American LGBTQ+ discourse. It offers a progressivist vision when it sutures itself to the perspective of the two, but not when it collapses into the position of the multiple. Thus, when it proliferates 'one' identity alongside another identity, it runs the risk of accelerating the process of identity formation and introducing subjects who are no longer dupes of the unconscious, and who might will for themselves certain identities (without recognizing that a considerable part of the self, of the *ego*, is submerged within the unconscious). We should ask ourselves what the function of the 'plus' is within the acronym LGTBQ+. Is it an attempt to remove oneself from the exception by affirming this exception as already included within the reign of the universal epistemological designation? What is shown in Figure 7.1 is how LGBTQ+ discourse might sometimes attempt to *say it all* about the sexed body.

Incidentally, each time we return to the positions, theories, and concepts already discussed (each time we cite them), we also change them, develop them, and twist them into new and interesting directions. This was also the promise of the perspective of the two: to no longer remain blind to the citational practices but to become aware of their truth procedures and to recognize that we are in fact duped by them.

A Mobius strip (Figure 7.2) might be produced by taking a thin rectangular sheet of paper, which, in the beginning consists of two

(+) Identity (-) Language

	Paradigm	Theories	Concepts
1.	Essentialist		
		Trumpian	Birth/Biology
		1st Wave feminist	Pay equity, Vote
2.	Social constructionist		
		Classical Marxist feminism	Ideology, Exploitation, Surplus value
		Intersectionality	Matrix of domination, Situated knowledge
		Queer theory	Citational practices, Performativity

(-) Identity (+) Language

Figure 7.1 Altered simplified chart

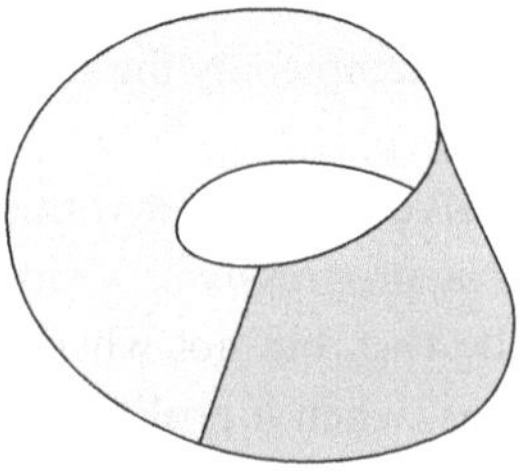

Figure 7.2 Mobius strip

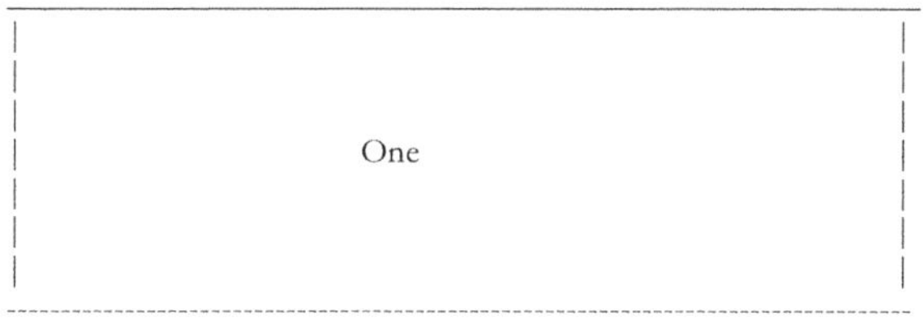

Figure 7.3 Surface one

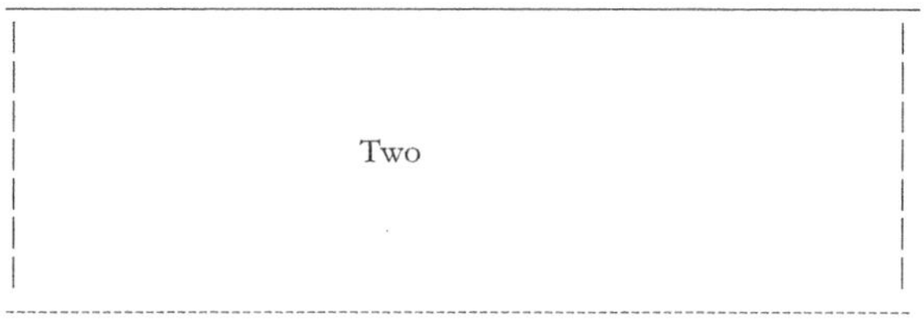

Figure 7.4 Surface two

surfaces (*recto* and *verso*), and bringing the short edge around, twisting it 180 degrees, and connecting it to the other short edge. In this way, the perspective of the one and two are brought together into a continuous surface. Although the perspective of the 'one' and 'two' are distinct they are nonetheless continuous with one another. Admittedly, this is a difficult idea to grasp: how can they be distinct and continuous at the same time? It is only by visualizing the Mobius strip that we can begin to understand that apparent paradox. We begin with a rectangular surface, and we write upon that surface the word 'one,' as shown in Figure 7.3.

This is now the *recto* side. But we can flip the rectangle over and write on the *verso* side the word 'two,' as shown in Figure 7.4.

Currently, there is a single sheet of paper with two surfaces: 'one' and 'two,' representing, respectively, the 'essentialist' and 'social constructionist' paradigms. It is not coincidental that the perspective of the two is on the obverse side of the sheet of paper: it is hidden from the perspective of the one, but nonetheless present and dependent upon it. When we are in the perspective of the one, we by definition ignore that there is another side to the sheet of paper. We take the surface we are on for granted without realizing that its support is a hidden secondary surface.

We shall see that this analogy can bring us very far in understanding American gender theory. We should take the word *verso* in the following sense: it is not just the obverse side of the sheet of paper, it is also a 'turn' upon the *recto* side. We should be reminded of the work of Georg Simmel, a classical German sociologist, who put forward an approach within sociology named 'social geometry.' His strategy was to look at the various spatial relations that exist within social bonds. For example, in his "Quantitative Aspects of the Group" (1950), he introduced the social geometry of the dyadic and triadic social groups. Although the sociological school of 'symbolic interactionism,' appropriately named by the American sociologist Herbert Blumer, has attempted to have the last word on Georg Simmel's work, it is not the case that he fits very neatly into its precepts. For example, it is clear that Simmel was engaged in a geometry or topology when he discusses the relationship of the elements within a set of individuals and those outside:

> [S]ociological formations . . . depend upon the numerical determination of their elements. In the case of dyads and triads, the point at issue was the inner group life with all its differentiations, syntheses and antitheses, as it develops at those minimum or maximum numbers of members. The concern was not with the group as a whole in its relation to other groups or to a larger group of which it is a part, but rather with the immanent mutual relationship among its elements. But we may also ask the inverse question regarding the significance of numerical determination for the relations of the group with the outside.
>
> (Simmel, 1950: 169)

What we discover is the following: a group with only two members is without secrecy for no other reason than because of the proximity and intimacy of the bond. Distance is lacking between members; they are fused together into a volatile union not unlike the sort of fusion one would expect between a mother and her newborn child. This is a fragile bond precisely because of its lack of distance: if one person is removed from the bond, then the entire group has disintegrated. However, if another member is added to the group then the distance between any two members is achieved because of the mediation of a third. Suddenly, alliances and secrecy shall develop, and one member may become a stranger to the bond by being pushed toward its periphery. The stranger is therefore 'in the group but not of the group,' which means, in other words, he is on the periphery of the group and therefore less anchored to its modes of self-identification.

Within our simple chart there are two vectors, one of which is related to the concept of identity. And we can see, from the vantage point of the two, that the concept of identity is more anchored to the perspective of the one. This is what the plus indicates. Thus, a vector exists, extending from the first perspective to the second perspective. The 'plus' and 'minus' indicate only that there is more or less of a fixation to the principle of identity. Whereas the first perspective remains fixed because identity is endlessly unexamined, in the second perspective it is by discovering the concept of identity that one paradoxically has found a space outside of it. We might draw one of these vectors in another way, as shown in Figure 7.5.

The concept of identity exists on the vertex of the perspective of the one. We should presume that it is present and that it is taken for granted, and then, as we move from that point of departure on the newly established vector, we also move, consequently, toward a possible political position. Thus, on second adjoining vertex there is a

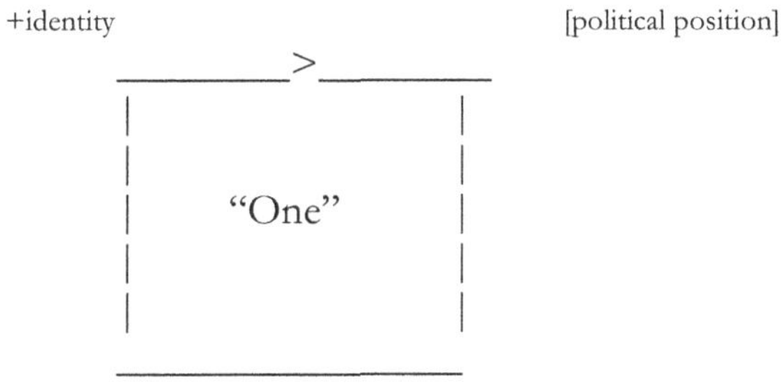

Figure 7.5 Surface one, first vector

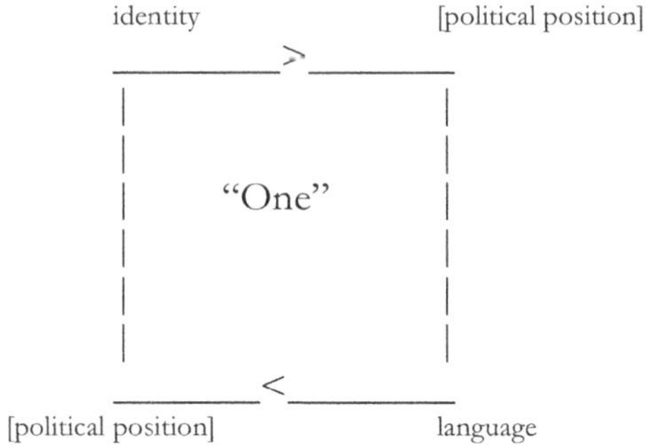

Figure 7.6 Surface one, two vectors

political position. Yet on the other side of the simple chart there was another possible vector: language. Whereas identity was a truth procedure discovered by the social constructionist perspective to be dormant within the essentialist perspective, language is an innovation of the social constructionist perspective used to analyze the citational practices of essentialism. Moreover, this perspective has found that identity is itself built upon the citational practices of language. For this reason, we can plot another vector on the perspective of the one, as in Figure 7.6.

Language exists on the opposite corner of the surface because it is opposed to the concept of identity even while it is its support. It is by emphasizing the role of language that we can situate ourselves partially outside of identity, precisely by recognizing ourselves subjected to linguistry. The emphasis on language also exposes the zone of conflict: there is the language of male versus female, proletarian versus bourgeoisie, and so on. We use language to give expression to these conflicts, and this is why it is only after passing through the vector of language that we can begin to approach the perspective of the two (which has an inherent emphasis on conflict and contradictions). We are led, then, to a different political position. In summary: we have two vertices ('identity' and 'language') and two consequences, represented abstractly by two different political positions, respectively: 'reactionary' and 'progressive.'

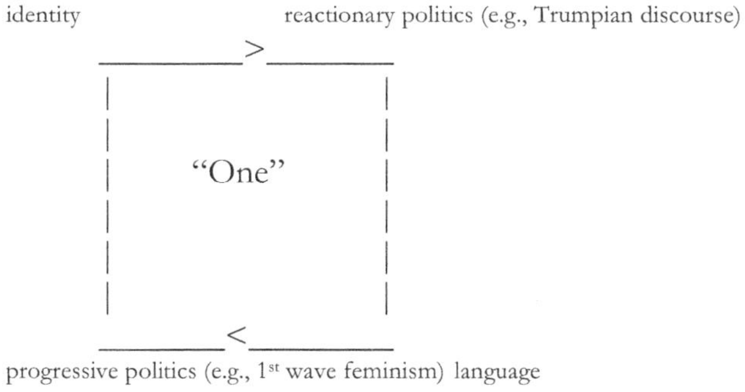

Figure 7.7 Surface one, full figure

When we begin from the blind acceptance of the concept of identity (rather than the position that linguistry gives rise to this concept), then we by necessity move toward a type of reactionary essentialism. This is the position of Trumpian discourse. The progressive position begins with the assumption that language and conflict are important for sustaining politics, and so it leads us to the theories of the first wave feminists (which are a sort of progressive essentialism for the time), as shown in Figure 7.7.

Progressive essentialisms move reflexively through the concept of identity. It is by deploying the concepts of pay equity, suffrage, and so on, that one is able to expose the rift that not only separates the genders but produces problematic distributions of wealth and power. Thus, progressive essentialisms reflect upon and return to the concept of identity but from within the domain of language.

As shown in Figure 7.8, we have the following two vectors: one that moves from the concept of identity to reactionary politics, and one that moves from the concept of language toward that of reactionary politics. Whereas the former vector signals a universalist conviction, the latter begins to articulate an exception; the former implies that identity is universal, and the latter implies that there are exceptions to this rule: some identities are excluded from universal humanity. The universal declaration consists of proclaiming that all men are to be treated equally or that all men and women are defined by their

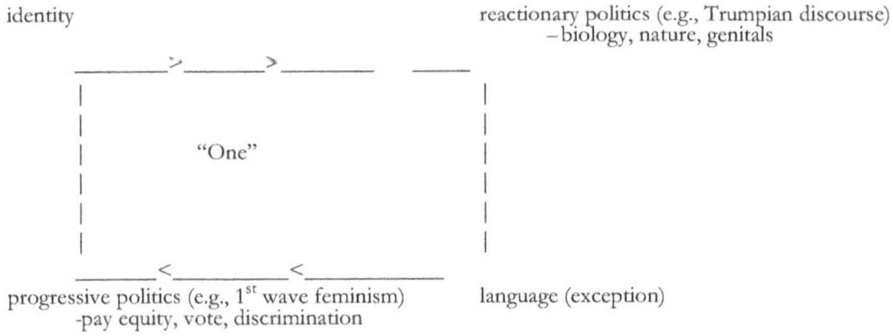

<u>Vectors</u>: → UNIVERSAL [identity is universal]
← EXCEPTION [men and women are treated differently; women are an exception to the universality of "human"]

Figure 7.8 Surface one with vector labels

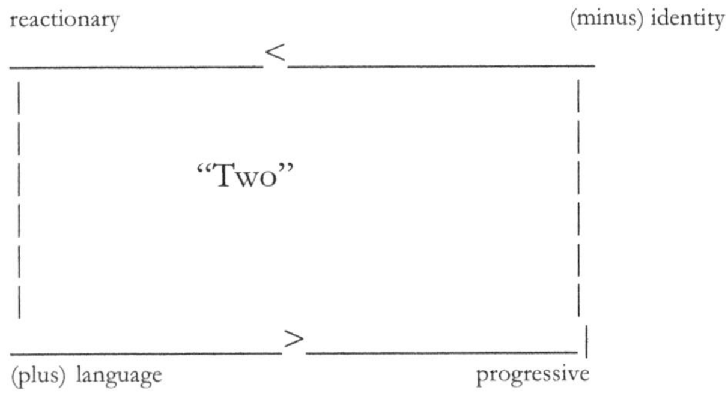

Figure 7.9 Surface two, two vectors

biological markers. The exceptional declaration consists of proclaiming that universal humanity consists primarily of men (and this misses the biological marker of the feminine).

On the obverse side, there is the perspective of the two. The already established vectors are inverted, and the result looks like what is shown in Figure 7.9.

In this case, we begin with the vertex on the top right: there is a problem with the concept of identity for thinking about gender (indicated by the minus). We are trying to move away from any position

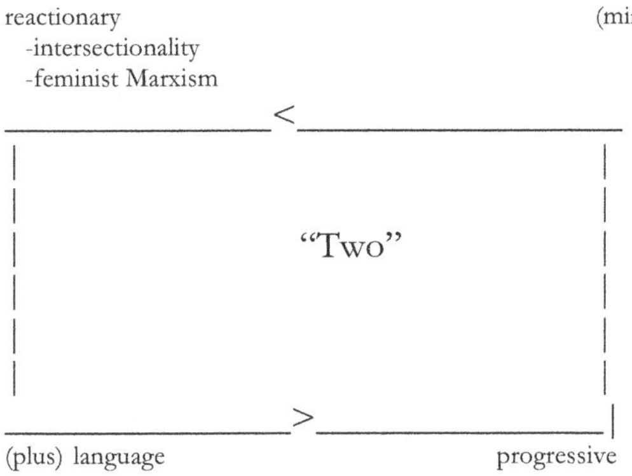

Figure 7.10 Surface two, full figures

that takes for granted established gender identities. On this surface, we are trying to demonstrate that identity always eclipses the multiplicity of situated identities. From within the paradigm of social constructionism, intersectionality and feminist Marxism therefore become politically reactionary, as shown in Figure 7.10.

Some readers will be disappointed in me for situating intersectionality and classical Marxist feminism within the reactionary political type. However, it is not meant as a normative judgment but rather as an awareness of its situatedness with respect to the concept of identity upon the surface of its paradigm. From the perspective of the one, intersectionality and Marxist feminisms are certainly progressive, but they are not any more progressive from the perspective of the two. If we begin by working ourselves out of the concept of identity (e.g., the mandate of the perspective of the two), then we take as our point of departure 'minus-identity.' If we follow this vector, then we begin by affirming an endless assortment of ones and regress into the 'multiple.'

Reactionary politics consists of an attempt to work two-selves out of the concept of identity only by affirming all the more *identities*, or one-selves. Thus, the perspective of the 'multiple' is simply a return to the perspective of the one, pluralized: it is a multiplicity of ones. Whereas 'intersectionality' consists of a progressive attack upon *the* first wave feminist movement, it is nonetheless a regressive operation when it works itself out of identity as such. Similarly, Marxist feminisms were progressive attacks upon the essentialist underpinnings of classical Marxist theory, but they nonetheless remain sutured to a fundamental identitarian position. For this reason, we combine the two surfaces into a continuous one by placing the progressive vector into the reactionary of the preceding side. What is reactionary for the one surface may transform into progressive on the other surface, and vice versa.

When we begin with an emphasis on the centrality of language (for the construction of identity, and so on) we are much closer to the position of queer theory. This is why we place queer theory at the apex of the perspective of the two, as shown in Figure 7.11: it affirms, more than any other position within social constructionist thought, the citational practices involved in gender identity.

Here, once again, we have two vectors defined by universality and exception. However, this is a different type of universality and exception than the one found in the perspective of the one. The vector of exception is this time at the top of the surface, and the exception gives rise to the proliferation of identities. Thus, we witness here within the perspective of the two the exception to the concept of identity in the form of multiplicities. On the bottom edge there is the negative

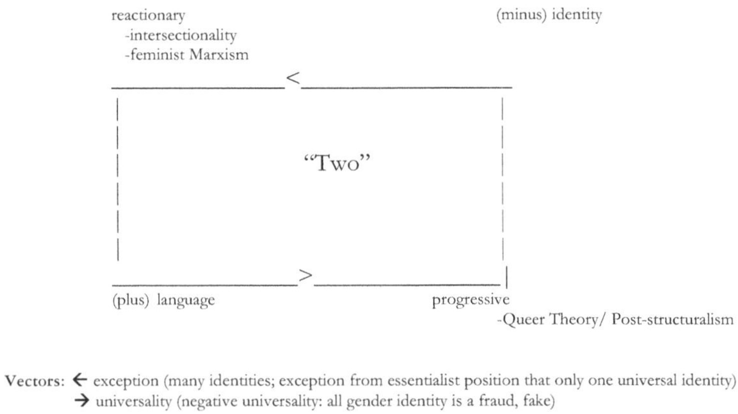

Figure 7.11 Surface two with vector labels

universality which, in its progressive form, proclaims not merely that language is the only game in town but rather that it is precisely because language is the only game in town that *all gender identity is a fraud*. Thus, the progressive position of queer theory, found in genderqueer is not the fluidity of gender but rather the fraudulence of gender as a linguistic construction.

The reader will at this point notice that I have not at all fleshed out all of the various theories that exist within gender studies or within the sociology of gender, nor have I introduced all of the various nuances of the theories. It is not my intention to do so, it is rather my intention to expose only those crucial nodal points that are useful for our topological study of American gender theory. This has allowed us to count to two, but it does not yet permit us to count to three. It is my intention now to begin to open up the perspective of the three, or what, for lack of a better term, I name the 'psychoanalytic paradigm.'

We have for the first time within the perspective of the two the position that gender exists within the category of sex, such that we require two terms to fully engage with any identity attributed to the sexed body. There is the 'biological facticity of the body' and there is gender as an inherited social script. This perspective proposes that *Sex != Gender*. Sex does not equal gender, there is a lack of correspondence between the two. We could also introduce vectors to demonstrate the principal orientation of the paradigm. We have the following two perspectives, then:

1 Sex == Gender
2 Sex ← Gender

Minimally, the way to read this formula is as follows: gender 'interprets' the sexed body. In the second perspective the sexed body is something that exists independent of and radically outside of language. Gender exists only in its function of interpreting the material reality of the body; or rather, gender *is the material reality of the body itself* since language can also be said to have a materiality. In other words, gender interprets the body, but it does so always against a hard limit, and this hard limit is the sexed body. As such, gender can never *say it all* about sex. The psychoanalytic position, put forward by

Alenka Zupancic (2017), Marie-Helene Brousse (2019), and others, is that sex, as a hole or fundamental impossibility within symbolic and imaginary frameworks, is also a force that operates upon those frameworks. It is this position that the social constructionist cannot understand, *literally*.

We have three paradigms, then:

1 Essentialist: Sex == Gender

2 Social constructionist: Sex ← Gender

3 Psychoanalytic:
←
Sex Gender
→

The psychoanalytic paradigm introduces another presupposition within the paradigm, which precedes it while also drawing out its inherent implications. This is why in order to have two, you must first have three. It is true that gender interprets the biological facticity of sex (left vector) but it is also true that sex introduces a fundamental impossibility for gender interpretations (right vector). Moreover, it is possible that it is because of the impossibility of sex (e.g., the impossibility of writing sex, of writing the real sexed body) that gender itself has its linguistic power. Gender does not have the last word on sex because there is no last word possible: from within the finite system of language, it is always possible to say something else, but this infinity is only possible within the finite system of language itself. Infinity is here put to the service of the finite system of language.

Gender interprets sex. Sex interrupts, resists, disrupts gender. The right vector moving from sex to gender implies interruption. Clinical psychoanalysts recognize this in their everyday practice. What they have realized, since the time of Sigmund Freud, is not that everything is reduced to a sexual meaning (since this implies that there is only a symbolic unconscious) but rather that sex disrupts every symbolic interpretation (this implies that there is a *real* unconscious). It is not therefore that sex is the site of some deeper meaning that has yet to be interpreted by the clinician. It is rather that we begin with too much fixation, too much meaning, and too many interpretations, and then we run up against the hard limit of castration anxiety. This, precisely, is what sex *means*. Something is missing from the symbolic apparatus itself.

Sex intrudes into our life as something that is beyond meaning, something that is at the limits of meaning, and something that throws us radically out of joint. The failure of gender is always the limit of sexuality. Whether progressive or reactionary, sex will always disrupt and distort our basic symbolic narratives and imaginary frameworks. The perspective of the 'third' engages with this missing dimension. The 'dumb' body fights back against language, against any social construction, against identity, without at all returning to the 'multiple,' and without at all affirming a 'one.' Not one, not two, but three.

References

Brousse, Marie-Helene. (2019) "The Black Hole of Sexual Difference," *The Lacanian Review Online*. As Retrieved on May 23rd, 2019 from <www.facebook.com/thelacanianreviewonline/>

Lacan, Jacques. (1973) *The Seminar of Jacques Lacan, Book XXI: Les Non-Dupes Errent*. As Retrieved on May 25th, 2019 from <www.valas.fr/IMG/pdf/THE-SEMINAR-OF-JACQUES-LACAN-XXI_les_non-dupes_errent.pdf>

Simmel, Georg. (1950) "Quantitative Aspects of the Group," in *The Sociology of Georg Simmel* (Kurt H. Wolf, Ed., Trans.). Glencoe, IL: The Free Press. pp. 87–174.

Zupancic, Alenka. (2017) *What Is Sex?* Cambridge, MA: MIT Press.

8 Subject formations

Part of my teaching strategy consists of demonstrating to my students the torment and torture of thinking. I do not arrive in the classroom with slides, or, as the Americans put it, 'modules,' but rather with some provisional formulae, scribbles, and so on. Thus, the student can expect to hear moments of silence, blunders, stuttering, and so on. I do not aim in the classroom to overcome the undesirable feeling of anxiety. I attempt to teach my students the value of Søren Kierkegaard's statement that "[w]hoever has learned to be anxious in the right way has learned the ultimate" (Kierkegaard, 1973: 139). However, we need to be very careful about this word 'learned,' since, in our case, we are not interested in learning as a manipulation of knowledge. We instead place the emphasis on the 'whoever,' that is, on the *subject* of the sentence.

A *subject* formation exists when there is anxiety, that is, when a subject is confronted by anxiety. For the moment, we might presume that there are two possible responses to the demands of anxiety: *fight* or *flight*. Those who run away from anxiety seal themselves off from its inherent possibilities; it is a flight from the new possibility toward the comfort of the situation that preceded it. It is an inherently reactionary subject formation, and truthfully, it is a cowardly one too. The reactionary subject formation is inherently cowardly because it exists only as a defence against the confrontation or irritation of anxiety. We might plot this in the following way:

1 Reactionary subject formation → cowardly → retreats from anxiety into a prior comfort

The second subject formation also seals itself off from anxiety, but by using a different technique. When the subject is faced with anxiety, there is a moment of haste: the subject runs quickly through the anxiety, to what appears to be its end point, toward that which appears to be a new comfort and a new mode of resolving the conflict. In this case, it is not that the subject enjoys the anxiety – although this possibility does also exist – but rather that the subject acts or thinks too quickly. This subject does not flee into a prior comfort but rushes toward an adequate or acceptable solution. Admittedly, this is a progressive subject formation, and so it is also a more courageous one. The progressive subject desires to move through the anxiety, to confront it, but in confronting it the problem is only renewed, or new problems are produced. The progressive subject contributes to the production of new difficulties, displacements of anxiety, new conflicts, and so on, and so only conceals the anxiety.

2 Progressive subject formation → courageous → acts in haste through the anxiety

Minimally, these are the two subject formations, and they are associated with reactionary and progressive political positions. Let us take as a simple example the study of hegemonic and hybrid masculinities. The concept of "hegemonic masculinity" was first put forward by Raewyn Connell in the 1980s (Connell, 1982, 1983), but it has taken on a number of different interpretations since that time. Much of the discussion I will now engage shall be reformulations of arguments also put forward by Messerschmidt and Messner (2018) and Bridges and Pascoe (2018) in relation to Connell's ideas. Originally, the concept of 'hegemonic masculinity' seemed to originate from within the perspective of the two to diagnose a form of essentialism: it described "fixed types of masculinity" (Messerschmidt & Messner, 2018). Otherwise, it was used to describe the dominant type of masculine discourse occurring within a particular historical moment and geographical location.

The following problem inevitably occurred: this definition was too restrictive because we soon came to realize that the dominant discourse on masculinity is not always hegemonic, and conversely, the non-dominant discourse on masculinity is not necessarily subversive.

It is not true that submerged discourses on masculinity are inherently progressive, therefore. Indeed, Messerschmidt and Messner found that this is not true for "bro culture," which, in its own way, only renews, in a reactionary way, hegemonic masculine discourse. It is therefore important to discover new criteria for distinguishing hegemonic and non-hegemonic masculinities. The way that Messerschmidt and Messner, as well as Bridges and Pascoe, have distinguished this was to argue that hegemonic discourses of masculinity are always those that aim to erase the essential conflict or anxiety inherent to gender (whereas non-hegemonic discourses are often attempts to point at and discuss those conflicts, inequalities, anxieties, and so on).

Connell does something particularly interesting by discussing "progressive and regressive social change in gender relations" (as cited by Messerschmidt & Messner, 2018: 36–7). I have resituated this sort of inquiry by asking: what, precisely, gives rise, at the level of discourse, to these two subject formations? If hegemonic masculinities are responsible for legitimating, through discourse, "unequal gender relations" (ibid.), then it does so always as a response to gender anxiety and conflict. When the subject is faced with anxiety, an opportunity presents itself to become 'complicit' or to 'protest.' Whereas in the former case the subject derives benefits and comforts from the hegemonic discourse, in the latter case the subject over-compensates by forming men's groups, exaggerating masculine stereotypes, and so on.

These two possibilities, rearticulated here but derived in essence from Connell, relate very well to the *reactionary* and *progressive* subject formations hitherto discussed. In the first case, the subject seeks comfort from the ensuing anxiety by retreating into the established discursive hegemony, and in the second case, the subject seeks to push the boundaries of the discourse in haste only to renew the stereotypical essence of masculinity. This latter formation is seen also in the figure of the hipster, whose flannel, beards, and so on, protest against dominant masculinity discourses.

A popular approach among sociological scholars of masculinity today is to focus on three levels of analysis:

1 Local (face-to-face, primary and secondary social groups)
2 Regional (country, state, institutional)
3 Global (international, media, world politics)

It is by producing these three levels or scales of analysis that one is able to demonstrate the fact that hegemonic masculine discourses can exist within any one level while non-hegemonic discourses could exist in another (Messerschmidt & Messner, 2018; Bridge & Pascoe, 2018). All of this is an indirect way of demonstrating the power of a simple definition: hegemonic masculinities are discourses aimed at erasing their status as discourses, which means that they aim at eradicating anxiety and erasing conflict. In other words, it does not matter what the scale of analysis is, whether local, regional, or global; all that matters is that the discourse occurs from the perspective of the one (or toward the perspective of the one from the perspective of the multiple). We have no reason to presume that submerged or marginalized discourses are inherently progressive or that the dominant discourse is somehow inherently regressive or reactionary. We require a more nuanced perspective, one that takes into account both the malleability of gender and the unavoidability of anxiety.

Bridges and Pascoe wrote that "gender is susceptible to extraordinary change; gender inequality is, by comparison, much more durable" (2018: 254). I would like to reorganize this passage into two sections. First, "gender is susceptible to extraordinary change" seems to me to be a statement that best encapsulates one of the axioms of queer theory: gender changes throughout time and across locations. However, this second section – "gender inequality is much more durable" – indicates a corrective or caveat: it implies that *although* gender is malleable it nonetheless retains an inherent conflict or anxiety. Gender anxiety becomes reproduced and rearticulated in ever new and deceptive forms.

We need to be willing to risk the possibility that subversive discourses can be used against us, transformed into hegemonic discourses, and so on. We should ever remain suspicious of any gender change by interrogating our various subject formations. It is possible that gender *itself* is the response of the subject to the anxiety of a "gender crisis" (Bridges & Pascoe, 2018). Moreover, it is possible that gender is itself a crisis of discourse, of language. Within discourse we run up against something that is *real*, something beyond language, such that we no longer know how to interpret the real sexed body. The result of any such crisis is by necessity a subject formation: cowardly or courageous. There are various subject formations, but I restrict myself for now only to these two, which might be plotted, provisionally, on our simple chart in the way shown in Figure 8.1.

There are, however, a few scales of analysis. For example, Trumpian discourse is reactionary and therefore cowardly (and the first wave feminist movement was progressive and therefore courageous). Yet taken together, the essentialist perspective is nonetheless a cowardly subject formation from the perspective of the more courageous social constructionist perspective. It is courageous from within the perspective of the one to be progressive and it is cowardly from the perspective of the two to retreat into the love of multiplicities. We therefore require new words to account for this difference of scale. I retain the 'cowardly' and 'courageous' distinction at the level of the paradigm, and I fall back upon the simple 'reactionary' and 'progressive' distinctions within the theoretical orientations, as demonstrated in Figure 8.2.

(Identity) (+) (-) Discourse Analysis

Paradigm	Theories
(1) Essentialist	Trumpian (reactionary) (cowardly) 1st wave (progressive) (courageous)
(2) Social Constructionist	Classical Marxist fem. (reactionary) (cowardly) Intersectionality Queer theory (progressive) (courageous)

(Identity) (-) (+) Discourse Analysis

Figure 8.1 Altered simplified chart

Paradigm	Theories	
(1) Essentialist	Trumpian → reactionary 1st wave → progressive	→ cowardly
(2) Social constructionist	Classical Marxist fem. → reactionary Intersectionality Queer theory → progressive	→ courageous

Figure 8.2 Paradigm with subject formulation

In any case, the various subject formations operate also through the figure of the 'metrosexual,' 'hipster,' and 'bro.' In each case there is what Bridges and Pascoe refer to as "selective borrowing" of non-hegemonic masculinities only to renew hegemonic discourse. For example, within 'bro' culture there is an attempt not to uncover the ways that language compels the subject but rather there is an attempt to produce and control language itself: 'brogurt,' 'broga,' 'brogrammers,' 'bromance,' 'brotein,' and so on. This linguistic practice is not an attempt to torture language to produce room for the subject, it is rather an attempt to manipulate language precisely to naively demonstrate that one is outside of its citational practices. It is an attempt to control the words that otherwise might have compelled us to think and act in accordance with hegemonic ideology.

This is what it means to walk along the Mobius strip: a progressive political position, one that might at one time appear courageous (i.e., holding hands with another man, acting or dressing a bit feminine) can in all actuality be quite cowardly and regressive. This is particularly apparent in the discourse of 'hybrid masculinity,' which refers to a

> [s]elective incorporation of elements of identity typically associated with various marginalized and subordinated masculinities and femininities (sometimes) into privileged men's gender performances and identities. These transformations include men's assimilation, among others, of 'bits and pieces' of identity projects coded as 'gay,' 'black,' or 'feminine.'
>
> (Bridges & Pascoe, 2018: 254)

The problem is that these hybrid masculinities are deceptive strategies meant to conceal unconscious conflicts and anxieties. It is precisely by appearing to overcome anxiety that one all the more renews it. Thus, I find myself in agreement with Bridges and Pascoe that "hybrid masculinity . . . simply shifts . . . the ways [power] systems are perpetuated," through the "preservation of gender conflict through transformation" (ibid.).

Thus, we have cowardly and courageous virtues, but perhaps what we require is, in all actuality, neither. Perhaps we require an intervention. When the subject feels gender anxiety, there is another strategy offered, which does not consist of fleeing or moving through it in haste. It is important to know how to make do with gender anxiety. An intervention *with* anxiety implies that one learns how to work through the anxiety. The perspective of the two often distances itself from the first perspective simply by adding more words to describe the gender conflict. Indeed, the social constructionists speak a lot: they write a lot of books, they teach a lot of courses, they are always forced to work through the problem of gender anxiety at the level of discourse itself. They are epistemologists who reject the agency of the body itself, who reject the real body and its real unconscious. And so they reject ontological considerations, ever suspicious of it for bearing the stamp of naïve essentialism.

Language *matters* for the perspective of the two. We now have the following three positions:

1 Sex == Gender (no language)
2 Sex ← Gender (language interprets)
3 Sex →
  ← Gender (language interprets; body resists/disrupts language)

For the third perspective, sex not only poses an obstacle to gender but in fact allows for something like gender to continue to produce ever further interpretations and scripts both historically and geographically. Thus, within the finite system of gender language there is, thanks to the real sexed body, the possibility of an infinite list of identities. The real sexed body is also an infinite source of determination for the linguistic possibility of gender itself.

In the last decade, queer theorists from the psychoanalytic orientation have begun to identify limitations within queer theories of gender and sexuality. They have begun to ask: "what comes after queer theory?" Or, put another way, what comes after post-structuralist and post-modernist scholarship within the field of the sociology of gender and sexuality? Are we capable of producing an intervention into the perspective of the two? We might reformulate our three perspectives in the following way:

1 Reactionary subject → cowardice → flees from gender anxiety
2 Progressive subject → courageous → hastes through gender anxiety
3 Sexed subject → courageous → accepts gender anxiety

It is possible that one day the word 'queer' will become acceptable for those in power. Perhaps it already has become integrated by reactionary subject formations, thereby obscuring gender anxieties and conflicts. Perhaps capitalism itself has become queer, as it supplements and seeks out avenues of liquidity. Zygmunt Bauman (2012) has claimed that we have entered an age of "liquid modernity" such that not only has "hard capital" has sought to seep through the cracks of the nation states, but epistemology itself has sought to seep through the cracks of any identity. At the same time, *the* queer has emerged as an acceptable identity formation, a 'one' within the great multiplicity of 'ones.' When we assert queer identities, we also risk losing ground on the fundamental insight of queer theory: linguistic determination as the prefiguration of identity. We exchange this insight for the more ideological one: that we are somehow capable of stepping outside of these scripts in order to produce identity configurations that no longer determine us.

This is why the position of the multiple is always a regress: it returns the subject to the concept of identity, to taken-for-granted constructs, under the guise of progressivism. These identities only reproduce and preserve gender anxiety and conflict. Indeed, some of today's queer theorists are now claiming that the concept of 'sexual identity' is a contradiction of terms (see Penney, 2014; Zupancic, 2017). If it is true that gender identity fixes meaning into a cultural sign, then sexual identity is a contradiction, since sex itself always resists being fixed. The sexed body is always a site of anxiety within *any* overarching gender script, and it does not matter which identity is asserted. Sex is perhaps nothing but the name we give for this hole within the linguistic determination of gender itself, while gender is often an attempt to tranquilize this anxiety.

James Penney (2014) has claimed that the political project of queer theory consists of a double gesture: on the one hand, it wishes to be a political intervention through its critique of identity, and yet on the other hand it also wants to erect itself as a discrete identity (e.g., "I am queer"). This contradictory gesture is not at all productive but in fact opens up the space for a possible political regress: what is most promising and critical about intersectionality and queer theory is its reflexive intervention into prevailing gender conceptions. If the queer theorists were once asking "what is [gender] identity?" or "what is *gender*?" then today the psychoanalytic community is asking "what is *sex*?" The psychoanalytic discourse shifts from an emphasis or theory about gender to an emphasis or theory about sex: from epistemology to the relationship of ontology and epistemology.

What we discover is that sex is like a window: you cannot see it directly and yet you look through it to see the world around you. Gender consists of markings scribbled upon the glass, which both obscure and reveal not the view but the fact of there being a window at all. Since every window is also a wall, sex is the real; it is the primary site of the obstacle or barrier itself. Alenka Zupancic writes that "in psychoanalysis, sex is above all a concept that formulates a persisting contradiction" (Zupancic, 2017: 3). And this contradiction is not what many suppose it to be: it is not a contradiction of man and woman, that is, a contradiction *between* the sexes. Rather, the contradiction exists within each or any gender category or identity itself. The psychoanalyst is not confined to the perspective of the one in claiming, as the first wave feminists did, that there is essentially a conflict between men and women, although that certainly exists as well. Rather, the psychoanalytic discourse moves further than the perspective of the one or two by claiming that the contradiction is inherent to gender itself.

The proliferation of gender identities only obscures, and in fact displaces, the fundamental problem of the inherent anxiety of gender itself. Sexual identity is a contradiction in terms because sex is not only irreducible to any identity, but it is in fact also disruptive of any identity. This is the lesson that psychoanalysis teaches us and that which Alenka Zupancic (2017) has made very clear in her work. The fact of the hole of sex is unsettling for gender and it has been so historically. Alenka Zupancic and Slavoj Zizek have provided us with an example of the lengths we will go to conceal the hole of sex. For example, the early painters of Adam and Eve within the Christian tradition did not know what to do about their naked bodies: they painted fig leaves covering not only the genitals but also the belly buttons. This strategy apparently helped to resolve the question of their sexual emergence and its impact upon the body.

Indeed, in Genesis, the sexual organs were covered up with a 'fig leaf.' However, the English translation reveals an important sentence: “Adam and Eve were both naked *and were not ashamed*.” My first mistake was to presume that the Hebrew word for ‘ashamed’ translated seamlessly into English. We are led to believe that Adam and Eve were both naked and were not embarrassed over the exposition of their sexual organs. It was only after they placed fig leaves over their genitals that they became embarrassed. Incidentally, the Hebrew word for ‘ashamed’ means ‘not being covered,’ and this therefore renders the previous presumption incorrect. The correct meaning seems to be that: “Adam and Eve were both naked and were not being not covered.”

The double negative ‘not being not’ obscures the passage considerably. But this obscuration is a productive one because it reveals precisely the role of sex and the real body from the perspective of gender. We never actually cover sex because sex itself is an obstacle to any covering: to *not be not covered*, or to *not be without covering*, implies that the impossibility of sex was exposed. In other words, they were for the first time confronted with gender anxiety because of the impossibility to cover the hole of sex with the fig leaves: on the contrary, the fig leaves *produced* the hole by revealing it. To my surprise, my reading was confirmed by Pope John Paul II (see West, 2019). Zupancic writes that “by covering up ‘the sexual,’ one always also – and perhaps primarily – covers up something else, something that is *not there* and which tends to raise some deep ambiguities” (Zupancic, 2017: 143). Gender is that which conceals the hole of sex, of the sexual, and of the sexed body.

Gender is therefore a clever way to cover up what was not there to begin with, and for no other reason than to produce the belief that there was something there already to cover! Is it not the case that by covering up the belly buttons of Adam and Eve they only renewed suspicions? Thus, in other words, the role of the fig leaves are meant to cover up the fact of the hole of sex, the fact of there being nothing in the first place. Sex is impossible in this sense, in that, it does not actually exist; it escapes the materializing practices of language and gender. The provocation of gender is also its profound intervention: sex is not *biological*, it is *real*; it is not an essential positive attribute there at the beginning (as adherents of the perspective of the ‘one’ maintain). It is not therefore that sex is a part of the symbolic unconscious that must be uncovered through delicate analytical interpretations. In the third perspective we can claim that it is a part of the real unconscious, which cannot be interpreted but rather poses an obstacle to any such interpretation while nonetheless providing us with the possibility of interpreting, endlessly interpreting.

The role of psychoanalysis is not to normalize underlying sexual perversities or to iron out the queer. Rather, the role of psychoanalysis is to demonstrate precisely that sex itself is the deeper and more difficult issue that not only throws us out of join, throws out lives into disarray, but also that which compels us to act and think at all in the world. In the perspective of the three, sex is an exception to any social construct. The psychoanalyst will agree with the social constructionist perspective in claiming that all identities are the result of citational practices, except, that is, for sex and the sexed body. But this does not mean that the psychoanalyst regresses into biological essentialisms: sex is not biological, natural, or essential. On the contrary, sex is disruptive, impossible, without existence. Sex refuses and resists scientific and biological epistemes while nonetheless giving rise to them.

Zupancic writes that "the ironic point is, of course, that for Freud, sexuality *was* the deeper and more difficult issue behind different sexual practices, innuendos, and meanings – that it was something inherently problematic, disruptive, rather than constructive of identities" (Zupancic, 2017: 6). This, I maintain, is the limitation and source of the social constructionist perspective. It is why before we can count to two, we must first have already known how to count to three – without knowing it. And it is why, before we can count to one, we have already known, somehow, how to count to three. Three precedes two and one. However, as we shall see in Chapter 9, one does not need to know how to count to three in order to count to four. One requires only the ability to invent.

References

Bauman, Zygmunt. (2012) *Liquid Modernity*. Cambridge, UK: Polity Press.

Bridges, Tristan, & Pascoe, C. J. (2018) "On the Elasticity of Gender Hegemony: Why Hybrid Masculinities Fail to Undermine Gender and Sexual Inequality," in *Gender Reckonings: New Social Theory and Research*

(James W. Messerschmidt, Michael A. Messner, Raewyn Connell, & Patricia Yancey Martin, Eds.). New York: New York University Press. pp. 254–274.
Connell, Raewyn. (1982) "Class, Patriarchy, and Sartre's Theory of Practice," *Theory and Society*, Vol. 11, No. 3: pp. 305–320.
Connell, Raewyn. (1983) *Which Way Is Up? Essays on Sex, Class, and Culture*. Sydney and Boston: Allen & Unwin.
Kierkegaard, Søren. (1973) *The Concept of Anxiety* (Walter Lowrie, Trans.). Princeton, NJ: Princeton University Press.
Messerschmidt, James W., & Messner, Michael A. (2018) "Hegemony, Nonhegemony, and 'New' Masculinities," in *Gender Reckonings: New Social Theory and Research* (James W. Messerschmidt, Michael A. Messner, Raewyn Connell, & Patricia Yancey Martin, Eds.). New York: New York University Press. pp. 35–56.
Penney, James. (2014) *After Queer Theory: The Limits of Sexual Politics*. London, UK: Pluto Press.
West, Christopher. (2019) "The Theology of the Body: An Education in Being Human," As Retrieved on May 28th, 2019 from <www3.nd.edu/~afreddos/courses/264/west2.htm>
Zupancic, Alenka. (2017) *What Is Sex?* Cambridge, MA: MIT Press.

9 Trans* inventions

From anxiety to certainty

For this chapter, I shall move in another direction by focusing on the prefix 'trans*,' which means, in other words, 'to move beyond' or 'to cross over.' The first question we should ask ourselves concerns what trans* crosses beyond? My aim in this chapter – like the preceding chapters – is not necessarily to review all of the literature and so become obsessed only with the practice of citational practices, but rather to situate trans* discourse in order to see how it advances our three perspectives. Where can trans* discourse be situated? However, to be clear, it is not clear, even to me, that I am making the correct moves. I am myself engaged in a movement of thought, and when thought moves, that is, when it crosses boundaries of paradigms, it sometimes has as its only recourse invention of a new possibility.

We confront the possibility of a pure invention. Indeed, we confront with most trans* discourses the invention of a certainty. I shall reproduce our simplified chart in Figure 9.1.

Before we move any further, we should realize that we are confronted already with a gap, with something missing: where is the third perspective? The first perspective was essentialist and it reduced gender to sex by bracketing out gender (language) as such. Gender does not always *matter* because language as a materializing force is rejected and so takes the discourse from behind. This is why we do not require the word 'gender,' and why we can write the first perspective in the following way:

1 Essentialist: Sex(Gender)

(+) Identity (-)Language

Paradigm	Theory
(1) Essentialist	Trumpism 1st Wave feminism
(2) Social constructionist	Intersectionality Queer theory

(-) Identity (+)Language

Figure 9.1 Simplified chart

The second perspective – social constructionism – claims only that gender actively interprets the sexed body, constructing it, materializing it. In a sense, it begins with an agreement with the essentialist perspective: there is a biological entity, there is a sexed body. However, this body exists as a 'dumb' body written and made intelligible by and through the social environment. Thus, Judith Butler claimed that there was the "biological facticity of the body" as well as gender as an inherited script performed regularly as a means to inculcate gender as a cultural sign. We write the formula for this second perspective in the following way:

2 Sex $\leftarrow$ Gender

The third perspective claims that sex disrupts and confuses gender, sex is a hole within the epistemological mechanism of gender performativity itself. Thus, the sexed body exists in some real dimension outside of (and within) language, and this is a continual source of anxiety for the social environment, for the big Other, for language, and indeed, for subjects in their everyday lives. It is not only that sexual identity is a contradiction in terms (and I would add that gender identity is a redundancy) but rather that sexual orientations are always built upon a fundamental disorienting force of sexuality. Any sexual orientation is disturbed and can only be an attempt to feel one's way around in the dark continent of sex itself. We write this third perspective in the following way:

3 Sex ←
→ Gender

Each perspective – one, two, and three – introduces something essential for our study of gender and sex. We have the following truth productions, as outlined in Table 9.1.

In the first perspective, we witness the production of a gender identity: 'male,' and/or 'female.' It is the concept of identity itself that is produced within this paradigm, and it is a discovery that is made use of in the paradigms that follow. The discovery is that there is something within gender that remains the same, relatively speaking, and that this sameness fixes meaning for the sexed body. Social constructionism discovers that the truth concerns language; whereby truth is understood as always 'half said' by a paradigm, which means that it is never directly acknowledged although it nonetheless forms the truth of the paradigm. It finds language at the core of any gender identity. This is why we can draw an arrow, retroactively, toward the first perspective. The social constructionist paradigm also provides us with a new emphasis, a new production,

Table 9.1 Truth productions

Production		*Truth*
	1 Essentialist	
Identity		Language
	2 Social constructionist	
Language		Barrier
	3 Psychoanalytic	
Barrier		Invention
	4 Trans*	

and this is the material with which it works. It is the same material found to be the support of the paradigm which preceded it: language.

In each case, there is a *production* and there is a *truth*. And, when taken together, we have the following *truth productions:* identity, language, barrier, and invention. The first two truth productions were articulated in our Mobius strip and in the simple chart of the previous chapters. What we discovered in the perspective of the three, the psychoanalytic perspective, was that the social constructionist perspective also produces a truth that it refuses nonetheless to acknowledge: sex as a barrier or disruption. It finds that the social constructionist emphasis on truth is its most powerful production, and it makes it the center of its own paradigm (rather than the concept of identity). It attacks language as such, then: what are the limitations of language and of social scripts? The sexed body is an epistemological limitation, it exists at the point where the ontological reality of the body intersects with its epistemological justification. All of this forms the hidden truth of the second perspective.

However, now we have the added perspective of four: trans*. This complicates our model considerably. What trans* demonstrates is precisely that the barrier of sex, of the sexed body, discussed at length by psychoanalytic discourse, itself can be crossed. We can in fact cross the Rubicon of the sexed body. When Julius Caesar led his army across the shallow river separating Rome from Italy, when he broke the law, it caused a civil war that introduced entirely new forms of suffering. Similarly, when the Rubicon of the sexual barrier has been crossed, when language itself digs into the real body in order to change and reconfigure it, there are nonetheless news forms of suffering. The question is not whether or not one makes the choice to cross – since this would imply a normative judgment – but rather the following: what happens when the barrier is crossed? It is possible that a new truth is produced.

The fourth perspective seems to demonstrate that it is possible for gender to become equal to sex: *Gender == Sex*. However, this is to be distinguished from the essentialist perspective that places sex as equal to gender: *Sex == Gender*. However, this algebra implies a symmetry in the two positions. The two positions are distinguished on the basis of their inventions. Thus, I write, for the fourth perspective: *Gender(Sex)*. This gives us the following four perspectives:

1 Essentialist: Sex(Gender)
2 Social constructionist: Sex ← Gender
3 Psychoanalytic: Sex ← → Gender
4 Trans*: Gender(Sex)

It is clear that the fourth perspective does not begin with the assumption that sex is a disruption. Yet, this does not imply that there is an ideological mystification precisely because the underlying gender anxiety seems to have been replaced by a new form of suffering. Within the essentialist perspective, the biological body refused to accept that it was determined by language, and so found itself trapped within the arrogance of affirming blindly an identity. But within trans* perspectives, the body is changed by the gendered scripts, quite consciously. Identity is therefore produced rather than determined, and its logic is not one of ideology but rather one of pure invention. Language intervenes to change the body itself: this is why trans* discovers that the barrier can be crossed, and that moreover, it is through invention that sex as a hole was produced in the first place.

The biological body becomes invented as a consequence of the certainty of gendered language, gendered scripts, and this, precisely, is the profound invention of the subject formation. This is different from the first perspective because trans* perspectives do not claim that the sexed and biological body are unchanging and fixed. On the contrary, they demonstrate that the body *can be changed*. It is also different from the second perspective because trans* perspectives do not presume that gendered scripts merely interpret the sexed body and that our task is to work ourselves out of identity formations. Quite the opposite: trans* affirms identity as such, without complexifying it into pluralities. Rather, a single identity is affirmed with certainty. Trans* is in some ways the triumph of the social environment, of language, over the sexed body, and through the willingness of the subject formation to be certain about this move, it indicates a new

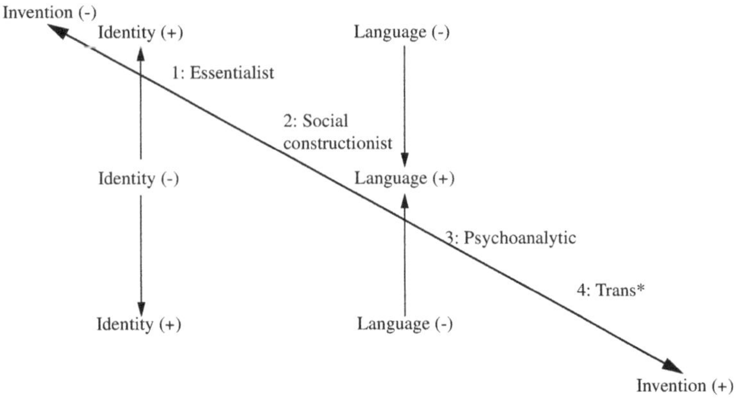

Figure 9.2 Completed chart

form of subjectivity. Yet it is not a triumph over the *subject*! This is the mistake that many psychoanalysts make.

The two new perspectives urges us to reconsider the simplified chart so that we might account for the new truth productions of 'barrier' and 'invention.' The new chart looks like what is shown in Figure 9.2.

Whereas the preliminary truth productions require only an 'x' and 'y' axis, for a surface that will be manipulated to produce a Mobius strip, the final two productions require another axis, the 'z' axis, which denotes, in Figure 9.2, the 'axis of invention.' Invention can come in many forms, but in its purest sense it occurs within trans* perspectives. More modestly, an invention can occur when, from within a given paradigm, one discovers something new. And each perspective discovers for itself a truth for that which preceded it (except the perspective of the one):

Truth productions

1 Identity → it is possible to have an identity
2 Language → it is possible that language determines identity
3 Barrier → it is possible that there is a barrier within language
4 Invention → it is possible to invent beyond a barrier

We therefore move from less inventive to more inventive as we move from the first perspective to the last perspective. For example, within the perspective of the one: first wave feminism invented the possibility that there is an inequality between the biological sexes within society; within the perspective of the two: queer theory invented the possibility that language torments the sexed body; within the perspective of the three: psychoanalysis invented the possibility that we should adopt an appropriate subject formation to accept the barrier of sex; and within the perspective of the four: trans* invented the possibility of crossing the barrier to invent the real body itself.

There is another interesting movement. As we move from psychoanalytic to trans* perspectives, there is a movement back to the concept of identity. Whereas one once worked oneself out of the concept of identity, one now returns to it, in a new way and inventive manner. After queer theory the concept of identity becomes of increasing significance. Identity, for trans* discourse, is no longer a site of suffering but rather a site of stabilization and healing. For this reason, the determining force of language becomes diminished as one approaches the fourth perspective. For trans* perspectives, language is no longer that which merely interprets the sexed body, but it is that from which one might derive, finally, a sense of certainty. Whereas essentialist perspectives were interested in identity but rejected language, trans* uses language not as an obstacle or barrier to gender but rather as that which supports identity.

Finally, we should comment upon this final possible subject formation. We have until now been discussing subject formations as responses to gender anxiety. Invention, though, is a type of certainty that does not reject language but rather moves with it into and across the barrier of sex. Thus, we should properly plot these differences, as in Table 9.2.

The essentialist perspective demonstrates sex certainty, but one that is radically without invention. Thus, the first perspectives introduce productions without inventions, because properly speaking, there is a reluctance to examine the procedure of truth. Trumpism is a reactionary position that does not invent anything new but rather falls back into prior understandings of the sexed body. By contrast,

Table 9.2 Gender certainty and gender confusion in four paradigms

Gender certainty	*Gender confusion*
Essentialist:	Social constructionist:
Sex(Gender)	*Sex* ← *Gender*
Trans*:	Psychoanalytic:
Gender(Sex)	←
	Sex *Gender*
	→

a small invention occurs within the first wave feminist movement based upon the discovery that men and women are differently situated within the political, economic, and cultural dimensions of society. Trans* perspectives also introduce certainty. Trans* people are often certain of their gender and this certainty moves them toward an invention of the body. The sexed body must be made to conform with the certainty of the script. Thus, one might expect to find (though this is by no means meant to be exemplary of the trans* perspective) such statements as: "I *am* this gender, and I just need to bring my body into conformity." Whether essentialist or trans*, there are two modes of certainty.

It is this certainty that can cause problems for the subject. Subjects are capable of suffering from their certainty just as much as they are capable of suffering from their anxieties regarding doubt. It is the inability to bring the real body into conformity with the linguistic vision that causes suffering in the fourth perspective. It is an inability, in other words, to invent. It is only by exploring the scope and direction of certainty that clinicians see suffering possibly diminish. On the other side of the chart, there is a suffering that results from gender confusion rather than gender certainty. The social constructionist and psychoanalytic perspectives are often responses to gender confusion or gender troubles. In this case, the problem is that we cannot often live up to the gender that was assigned at birth. Identity is often a posturing or masquerade, and so we are forced to ask such foundational questions as "what does it really mean to be a man?" or "what does it really mean to be a woman?" and so on. The sexed body confuses us at the level of gender.

This is what it means to count to four. I do not imagine that America is yet prepared to count to five within gender theoretical discussions. We shall be lucky if we find ourselves prepared to count to two. It is not our task to make gender great again, it is our task to make gender count again.

Index

For Product Safety Concerns and Information please contact our EU representative GPSR@taylorandfrancis.com Taylor & Francis Verlag GmbH, Kaufingerstraße 24, 80331 München, Germany

Printed and bound by CPI Group (UK) Ltd, Croydon, CR0 4YY
14/09/2026
02216256-0002